SEPTIC SHOCK:
CURRENT PATHOGENETIC CONCEPTS, OPTIMAL MANAGEMENT, AND FUTURE PERSPECTIVES

Septic Shock:
Current Pathogenetic Concepts, Optimal Management, and Future Perspectives

George H. Sakorafas
and
Adelais G. Tsiotou

Nova Science Publishers, Inc.
New York

Library of Congress Cataloging-in-Publication Data
Available upon request

ISBN 1-59454-168-X

Published by Nova Science Publishers, Inc. ✢ New York

Contents

Preface

Sepsis is one of the most frequent complications in the surgical patient and one of the leading causes of mortality in intensive care units. During the past two decades, a great deal has been learned about surgical bacteriology, antibiotic prophylaxis, supportive management, and the host response to microbial invasion. Sepsis can be caused by infection with gram-negative bacteria, gram-positive bacteria, fungi (and particularly Candida), or viruses. Sepsis may also occur in the absence of detectable bacterial invasion, and in these cases, microbial toxins, particularly gram-negative bacterial endotoxin (lipopolysaccharide, LPS), and endogenous cytokine production have been implicated as initiators and mediators. Although activation of the immune system during microbial invasion is generally protective, septic shock develops in a significant number of patients as a consequence of a poorly regulated immune response to the offending organism. Sepsis can be presented with a spectrum of severity. Septic shock represents the most severe form of host response to infection. The aim of this monograph is to summarize the currently available data regarding epidemiology, pathogenesis, and optimal management of septic shock, with a particular emphasis on the role of source control in sepsis. Emerging therapies for septic shock are also discussed.

Chapter 1

Introduction

Sepsis is one of the most frequent complications in the surgical patient and one of the leading causes of mortality in intensive care units [1]. During the past two decades, a great deal has been learned about surgical bacteriology, antibiotic prophylaxis, supportive management, and the host response to microbial invasion. Sepsis can be caused by infection with gram-negative bacteria, gram-positive bacteria, fungi (and particularly Candida), or viruses. Sepsis may also occur in the absence of detectable bacterial invasion, and in these cases, microbial toxins, particularly gram-negative bacterial endotoxin (lipopolysaccharide, LPS), and endogenous cytokine production have been implicated as initiators and mediators [2, 3]. Although activation of the immune system during microbial invasion is generally protective, septic shock develops in a significant number of patients as a consequence of a poorly regulated immune response to the offending organism. Sepsis can be presented with a spectrum of severity. Septic shock represents the most severe form of host response to infection. The aim of this monograph is to summarize the currently available data regarding epidemiology, pathogenesis, and optimal management of septic shock, with a particular emphasis on the role of source control in sepsis. Emerging therapies of septic shock will also be discussed.

Definitions

Precise definitions are necessary to improve the ability to accurately diagnose, monitor, and treat septic patients. The 2001 International Sepsis

Definitions Conference,, held in Washington, DC, in December 2001, included 29 anticipants from Europe and North America [4]. The goals of this conference was "to provide a conceptual and a practical framework to define the systemic inflammatory response to infection, which is a progressive injurious process that falls under the generalized term "sepsis" and includes sepsis-associated organ dysfunction as well" [4]. The following entities have been described and defined in this conference:

SIRS

- The term "Systemic Inflammatory Response Syndrome" (SIRS) has been first introduced into common parlance during the 1991 ACCP (American College of Chest Physicians)/SCCM (Society of Critical Care Medicine) [5]. This syndrome is characterized by complex findings that result from a systemic activation of the innate immune response, regardless of cause (e.g., localized or generalized infection, trauma, thermal injury, sterile inflammatory disease process such as acute pancreatitis). SIRS is diagnosed when patients have more than one of the clinical findings reported at ***Table 1***.

Table 1. SIRS is considered to be present when patients have more than one of the following clinical findings

- body temperature $> 38^o$ C or $< 36^o$ C
- Heart rate > 90 / min
- Hyperventilation evidenced by a respiratory rate of > 20 / min or a P_aCO_2 of < 32 mm Hg
- White blood cell count of > 12000 cells / μL or < 4000 cells / μL

These criteria are nonspecific and therefore they can't be used to recognize a cause of the syndrome or to identify a distinct pattern of host response [6]. It should be emphasized that signs of systemic inflammation can be observed in the absence of an infectious cause of the syndrome. SIRS is associated with relatively consistent biochemical features, such as elevated circulating levels of IL-6 [7], adrenomedullin [8], soluble(s) CD14, sELAM-1, MIP-1[alpha] [9], extracellular phospholipase A2 [10], and C-reactive protein [11] in patients meeting the 1992 SIRS criteria. In the future it may be possible to use purely biochemical and/or immunologic, rather than clinical, criteria to identify the inflammatory response.

It may be that inflammation is present when the circulating concentration of IL-6, procalcitonin, or C-reactive protein is increased [12 - 14]. No large prospective studies currently support such a conclusion.

Sepsis

In 1992, sepsis was defined to the clinical syndrome characterized by the presence of both infection and a systemic inflammatory response (as a response to infection) [5]. The recognition of infection is important since effective therapies are available. The same definition has been adopted by the 2001 SCCM/ESICM/ACCP/ATS/SIS International Sepsis Definitions Conference [4]. The clinical manifestations would include two or more of the following conditions as a result of a documented infection:

- Body temperature higher than 38 ^{0} C or lower than 36 ^{0} C
- Heart rate higher than 90 / min
- Hyperventilation evidenced by respiratory rate higher than 20 / min or $PaCO_2$ lower than 32 mmHg
- White blood cell count higher than 12.000 cells/μl, lower than 4.000/μl, or > 10 % immature (band) forms

Infection

According to the 2001 International Sepsis Definitions Conference, infection has been defined as "the pathologic process caused by the invasion of normally sterile tissue or fluid or body cavity by pathogenic or potentially pathogenic microorganisms" [4]. Participants of this conference, however, recognized that this definition is not perfect. For example, colitis caused by Clostridium Difficile, results from overgrowth of this organism in the colon, which is certainly not sterile. Furthermore, the clinical manifestations of C. Difficile are not caused by the bacteria invading normally sterile tissues, but rather, by the cytopathic effects of an exotoxin secreted by the pathogen microorganism. It is also important to point out that, frequently, infection is strongly suspected without being microbiologically confirmed. Accordingly, sepsis (i.e. infection and the systemic response to it) may only be strongly suspected, without being microbiologically confirmed [4].

Table 2. Diagnostic criteria for sepsis

Infection [a], documented or suspected, and some of the following[b]:

General variables

- Fever (core temperature > 38.3 ^{0}C)
- Hypothermia (core temperature < 36 ^{0}C)
- Heart rate > 90 min^{-1} or > 2 SD above the normal value for age
- Tachypnea
- Altered mental status
- Significant edema or positive fluid balance (> 20 ml/kgr over 24 h)
- Hyperglycemia (plasma glucose > 120 mg/dL or 7.7 mmol/l) in the absence of diabetes

Inflammatory variables

- Leukocytosis (WBC count > 12.000 μL^{-1})
- Leukopenia (WBC count < 4000 μL^{-1})
- Normal WBC count with > 10 % immature forms
- Plasma C-reactive protein > 2 SD above the normal value
- Plasma procalcitonin > 2 SD above the normal value

Hemodynamic variables

- Arterial hypotension [b] (systolic blood pressure < 90 mm Hg, mean arterial pressure < 70, or a systolic blood pressure decrease > 40 m Hg in adults or < 2 SD below normal for age
- Mixed venous oxygen saturation ($S\nu O_2$) > 70 %
- Cardiac index > 3.5 $L.min^{-1}.\ m^{-2}$ [c,d]

Organ dysfunction variables

- Arterial hypoxemia (PaO_2 / FiO_2 < 300)
- Acute oliguria (urine output < 0.5 $mL.Kgr^{-1}.hr^{-1}$ or 45 mmol/L for at least 2 h)
- Creatinine increase > 0.5 mg/dL
- Coagulation abnormalities (INR > 1.5 or apt > 60 sec)
- Ileus (absent bowel sounds)
- Trombocytopenia (platelet count < 100.000 μL^{-1})
- Hyperbilirubinemia (plasma total bilirubin > 4 mg/dL or 70 mmol /L)

Tissue perfusion parameters

- Hyperlactatemia (> 3 mmol/L)
- Decreased capillary refill or mottling

WBC, white blood cell, INR, international normalized ratio

[a] Infection defined as a pathological process induced by a microorganism

[b] Values above 70 % are normal in children (normally, 75 – 80 %); therefore, NEITHER should be used as signs of sepsis in newborns or children

[c] Values of 3.5 – 5.5 are normal in children and should therefore not be used as a sign of sepsis in newborns or children

[d] Diagnostic criteria for sepsis in the pediatric population is signs and symptoms of inflammation plus infection with hyper- or hypothermia (rectal temperature > 38.5 ^{0}C or < 35 ^{o}C), tachycardia (may be absent in hypothermic patients), and at least one of the following indications of altered organ function: altered mental status, hypoxemia, elevated serum lactate level, and bounding pulses. From Ref # 4.

Systemic Inflammation in Response to Infection

Because of the limitations of SIRS discussed above, a list of possible signs of systemic inflammation in response to infection (i.e., sepsis) has been proposed (***Table 2***) [4]. This scheme seeks to codify the physical and laboratory findings that prompt an experienced clinician to conclude that an infected patient "looks septic". Findings indicative of early organ dysfunction may be the first symptoms noted by clinicians when making this assessment. It is for this reason that we included findings such as hemodynamic instability, arterial hypoxemia, oliguria, coagulopathy, and altered liver function tests among the list of criteria that can be used to establish the diagnosis for sepsis. It is important to emphasize that none of the findings reported in Table 2 is specific for sepsis; rather these changes can be observed in many other diseases/conditions, such as trauma or following major surgical procedures. In the "day-to-day" clinical practice, few, if any, patients in the early stages of the inflammatory response to infection are diagnosed with sepsis via four arbitrary criteria. Instead, the clinician, goes to the bedside, identifies myriad symptoms, and regardless of an evident infection, declares the patient to "look septic". If no obvious source of infection exists, the clinician then initiates a search for an infectious origin of signs and symptoms associated with sepsis.

Severe Sepsis (Sepsis with Organ Dysfunction)

The definition of severe sepsis remains unchanged and refers to sepsis complicated by organ dysfunction, tissue/organ hypoperfusion, or hypotention (***Tables 3 and 4***) [15, 16]. Severe sepsis is now considered to be the most common cause of death in non-coronary critical care units [17]. Organ dysfunction can be defined by using other definitions, such as those developed by Marshall et al [18] or by using the Sequential Organ Failure Assessment (SOFA) score [19]. Organ dysfunction in severe sepsis in the pediatric population can de defined using definitions developed by Wilkinson et al [20], Proulx et al [21], and Doughty et al [22]. Hypoperfusion and perfusion abnormalities may include, but are not limited to, lactic acidosis, oliguria, or an acute alteration in mental status.

Table 3. Definitions of organ failure

Cardiovascular failure.- Presence of one or more of the following:

- ✓ Heart rate ≤ 54 / min
- ✓ Mean arterial pressure ≤ 49 mm Hg (systolic blood pressure ≤ 60 mm Hg)
- ✓ Occurrence of ventricular tachycardia and/or ventricular fibrillation
- ✓ Serum pH ≤ 7.24 with a Pa_{CO2} of ≤ 40 mm Hg

Respiratory failure.- Presence of one or more of the following:

- ✓ Respiratory rate ≤ 5 / min or > 49 / min
- ✓ $Pa_{CO2} \geq 50$ mm Hg
- ✓ $(A - a)_{O2} \geq 350$ mm Hg $(A - a)_{O2} = 713\ F_{IO2} - Pa_{CO2} - Pa_{O2}$
- ✓ Depended on ventilator or CPAP on the 2nd day of OSF (i.e. not applicable for the initial 24 h of OSF)

Renal failure.- Presence of one or more of the following:

- ✓ Urine output ≤ 479 mL / 24 h or ≤ 159 mL / 8h
- ✓ Serum BUN ≥ 100 μgr / 100 mL (>36 μmol / L)
- ✓ Serum creatinine ≥ 3.5 μgr / 100 mL (> 310 μmol / L)

Hematologic failure.- Presence of one or more of the following:

- ✓ WBC ≤ 1000 μL
- ✓ Platelets ≤ 20.000 μL
- ✓ Hematocrit ≤ 20 %

Hepatic failure.- Presence of both of the following:

- ✓ Serum bilirubin > 6 mgr %
- ✓ Prothrombin time > 4s over control (in the absence of systemic anticoagulation)

Neurologic failure.-Glasgow Coma Score ≤ 6 (in the absence of sedation)

(From Ref # 15)

Septic Shock

Septic shock in adults refers to a state of acute respiratory failure characterized by persistent arterial hypotension unexplained by other causes. Hypotension is defined by a systolic arterial pressure < 90 mm Hg (in children < 2 SD below normal for their age), a MAP < 60, or a reduction in systolic blood pressure of > 40 mm Hg from baseline, despite adequate volume resuscitation, in the absence of other causes for hypotension.

Table 4. Common clinical and laboratory methods to evaluate specific organ system dysfunction

Respiratory dysfunction.

- ✓ Altered oxygenation status (decreased Pa_{O2}/Fi_{O2} or need for supplemental oxygen)

Renal dysfunction.

- ✓ Serum creatinine levels
- ✓ Urine output (especially oliguria)
- ✓ Need for dialysis

Hepatic dysfunction.

- ✓ Jaundice or hyperbilirubinemia
- ✓ Elevated serum transaminases, lactate dehydrogenase, alkaline phosphatase
- ✓ Hypoalbuminemia
- ✓ Elevated prothrombin time

Cardiovascular dysfunction.

- ✓ Hypotension,
- ✓ Arrhythmias
- ✓ Use of inotropic or vasopressor support
- ✓ Elevated central venous pressure or pulmonary capillary wedge pressure.

Hematologic dysfunction.

- ✓ Thrombocytopenia
- ✓ Leukocytosis or leukopenia
- ✓ Coagulopathy (elevated prothrombin time, partial thromboplastin time, fibrin degradation products, or other evidence of disseminated intravascular coagulation)

Gastrointestinal dysfunction.

- ✓ Gastrointestinal bleeding
- ✓ Acalculous cholecystitis
- ✓ Pancreatitis
- ✓ Ileus
- ✓ Intolerance of enteral nutritional support
- ✓ Intestinal ischemia or infarction
- ✓ Gastrointestinal perforation.

Neurologic dysfunction.

- ✓ Alterations in level of consciousness and cerebral function (decreased Glascow Coma Score)

Table 4. Continued

Endocrine dysfunction.
✓ Hyperglyceremia
✓ Hypertriglyceridemia
✓ Hypoalbuminemia
✓ Weight loss / hypercatabolism.
Immune system dysfunction.
✓ Hospital-acquired infections
✓ Pyrexia
✓ Increased leukocytosis
✓ Alterations in immune activity.

(From Ref # 16)

Children and neonates maintain higher vascular tone than adults. Therefore, the shock state occurs long before hypotension in children. Septic shock in pediatric patients is defined as a tachycardia (may be absent in the hypothermic patient) with signs of decreased perfusion including decreased peripheral pulses compared with central pulses, altered alertness, flash capillary refill or capillary refill < 2 sec, mottled or cool extremities, or decreased urine output [23]. Hypotension is a sign of late and decompensated shock in children.

It is important to emphasize that sepsis is a continuum of injury response, with increasing severity and mortality, ranging from sepsis to septic shock, to sepsis-induced multiple organ dysfunction syndrome (MODS) (i.e.. altered organ function in a acutely ill patient, such that homeostasis cannot be maintained without intervention).

Chapter 2

Epidemiology

Given the difficulty of prospectively identifying cases of sepsis on a large scale, Angus et al [17] used hospital discharge records from a single year from 7 states representing approximately 25 % of the total US population. They estimated that there were 750,000 cases of severe sepsis nationally in 1995, resulting in approximately 500 deaths per day. Similarly, other estimates reported more than 500.000 cases per year nationwide for the USA [3, 24]. The incidence continues to increase, but supporting data have been difficult to obtain because definitions have varied over time, between institutions and even among clinicians working in the same institution. Furthermore, sepsis is not a reportable disease, and this further complicates the estimation of the incidence and prevalence of this entity. The Centre for Disease Control (CDC) reported a dramatic 139 % increase in the incidence of sepsis over a recent 10-year interval [25]. In addition to the increase in incidence, there has been an increase in both gram-positive and gram-negative sepsis and a parallel increase in the mortality rate associated with sepsis [25, 26]. Factors that are potentially responsible for the growing incidence of sepsis and septic shock are an increased awareness and sensitivity for the diagnosis, an increased number of patients who have compromised immune status, the increased use of aggressive invasive procedures in patient management and diagnosis, a growing number of resistant microorganisms that are encountered in clinical settings, and an ever-growing number of elderly patients who are at greater risk for the development of sepsis and septic shock [24, 27].

Three recent European epidemiologic surveys were recently discussed at the 23rd International Symposium on Intensive Care and Emergency Medicine [28, 29]. The Scottish Intensive Care Audit Group (SICAG) study surveyed the incidence of intensive care unit (ICU)-specific diseases for a 5-month period throughout Scotland. On a larger scale, the SOAP study was performed as a multi-centre study across Europe over a period of 15 days. A similar study was conducted exclusively in France during a 2-week period (the Episepsis study). These studies observed differences in the rates of sepsis among European countries, including differences in common causative organisms. The occurrence of sepsis in the ICU was highest in the Scottish study, present in 46 % of all ICU patients at some point during their stay. Other surveys have documented sepsis to account for 2 – 5 % of all ICU admissions, and to occur in 5 – 25 % of all ICU patients. In comparing the French study with a previous similar study, the incidence of sepsis in the ICU appears to be rising, from the 9 % reported in the 1993 survey to 17 % now. An additional important finding is that 15 % of septic patients surveyed were still hospitalized for 2 months. Furthermore, among ICU patients with sepsis who ultimately die, 80 % will die while in the ICU.

Despite recent progress in antibiotics and critical care therapy, sepsis is still associated with a high mortality rate. Indeed, the outcome from this syndrome has not improved significantly in the past 40 years [30]. Epidemiological studies in both the United States and Europe showed that sepsis continues to have a high mortality rate (~ 40 - 50%), even when the infecting organism is known, appropriate antimicrobial therapy is administered, and state-of-the art intensive care facilities are provided [31 - 33]. The development of septic shock and sequential multiple organ failure / dysfunction syndrome (MOF/MODS) correlate with poor outcome, and septic shock is the most common cause of death in intensive care units [1 - 3]. Death from septic shock in the United States increased from 35.000 in 1970, to 94.000 in 1980, to 198.000 in 1990 [34]. The death rate from septic shock per 100.000 population increased from 1.7 in 1970 to 4.2 in 1980, to 7.9 in 1990 and to 7.9 in 1993 [34]. One quarter of the deaths result from complications directly attributable to the bacteraemia, whereas 10 % of the deaths are related to the underlying disease process [24]. In addition to the human cost of sepsis, recent figures state that sepsis accounts for $ 5 billion to $10 billion of the annual health care cost in the United States [35].

In a recent study, the ICU was the location of 59 % of the patients [1]. There were 2.0 episodes of sepsis per 100 hospital admissions or 2.8 episodes per 1000 patient-days [1]. Other studies have demonstrated incidence figures as low as 1.36 per 100 admissions or 1.06 per 1000 patient-days [36] and as high as 16 to 260 per 1000 patient-days [30]. ***Table 5*** summarises the risk factors associated with an increased risk for the development of sepsis and its complications. The recognition of these risk factors for sepsis may be useful for the clinician, since it might be possible to improve preoperative preparation and intervene in certain circumstances, therefore decreasing the risk of sepsis. However, if sepsis cannot be prevented, at least the prepared physician will recognize patients at an early stage and perhaps have a better chance of treating these patients [37].

Table 5. Factors associated with an increased risk for the development of sepsis

- Age < 3 and > 70 years
- Compromised immune status
  - ✓ Acquired immunodeficiency syndrome (AIDS)
  - ✓ Use of cytotoxic and immuno-suppressant agents (including steroids)
  - ✓ Severe malnutrition
  - ✓ Alcoholism
  - ✓ Malignancy
  - ✓ Diabetes mellitus (white blood cell dysfunction and impairment of phagocytosis)
  - ✓ Transplantation procedures
  - ✓ Cirrhosis (decreased hepatic reserve, inability to generate appropriate acute-phase proteins in response to sepsis).
  - ✓ Cardiovascular disease and chronic pulmonary disease (impaired oxygen delivery to the tissues and depressed bacterial killing)
  - ✓ Mixed connective-tissue disorders (impaired immune function).
  - ✓ Major trauma (depressed immune response).
  - ✓ Major elective operations (such as abdominal vascular procedures, hepatobiliary procedures, and large colon procedures) (impaired immune function)
  - ✓ Massive blood transfusions (causing immunosuppression).
- Inappropriate use of antibiotics (bacterial overgrowth, increased number or resistant microorganisms, and fungal sepsis).
- Failure of asepsis, particularly with the placement of multiple nosocomial devices (breakdown of host defenses).
- Liberal use of aggressive invasive procedures in patient management and diagnosis

Chapter 3

Pathophysiology of Septic Shock

The normal reaction to infection involves a series of complex immunologic processes. A potent, complex immunologic cascade ensures a prompt protective response to microbial invasion in humans. A deficient immunologic defence may allow infection to become established. However, an excessive or poorly regulated response may harm the host through a maladaptive release of endogenously generated inflammatory compounds. Sepsis results from an extensive triggering of the body's defence mechanisms by invading microorganisms (gram-positive organisms, fungi, and gram-negative organisms and their constituent endotoxins) or by extensive tissue injury, ischemia / reperfusion injury [38]. These defence mechanisms include the release of cytokines, the activation of neutrophils, monocytes, and microvascular endothelial cells, as well as the activation of neuroendocrine reflexes and plasma protein cascade systems, such as the complement system, the intrinsic (contact system) and extrinsic pathways of coagulation, and the fibrinolytic system. Therefore, sepsis is characterized by a generalized inflammatory response. The sepsis response may begin with an infectious nidus, which may either invade the blood stream, leading to dissemination and positive blood cultures, or proliferate locally and release various microbial products into the bloodstream. In multiple trauma or hemorrhagic shock, the direct tissue or secondary ischemia / reperfusion injury may also lead to an increased appearance of microorganisms and endotoxins from the gut. The host response to these microbial products or to the trauma and ischemia-reperfusion injury itself leads to the rapid activation of the innate immune response and the release of a variety of humoral mediators [38, 39]. All these inflammatory mediator systems become activated to some extent during sepsis. The interaction of these systems produces a microvascular injury that leads to organ / tissue ischemia and multiple organ dysfunction and / or failure [40, 41].

The Role of Macrophages

Macrophages represent the key recognition cell in the human host, since they are the first phagocytic cells to come in contact with the pathogens. Macrophages play a critical role in regulating the inflammatory response subsequent to an insult [42]. Central to this inflammatory process is the macrophage's ability to exert diverse cellular / intercellular effects and to release a number of cytokines. Profound alterations in macrophage population and function are common after severe stress and in patients with severe protein-calorie malnutrition (i.e., critically ill patients) [37]. As previously noted, the excessive, unregulated, prolonged stimulation of the macrophage (in conjunction with other active cells, such as leukocytes and the endothelial cells of the microvasculature) leads to a vicious cascade of inflammatory mediators release; these inflammatory mediators act synergistically to augment the inflammatory response [43, 44].

The Role of Neutrophils

Neutrophils produce a large number of agents (including proteases and toxic oxygen products) for the destruction of bacteria. Under normal conditions, little interaction occurs between neutrophils and the endothelium. However, they act in a nonspecific fashion and - when activated systemically or when the endothelium is activated by cytokines- neutrophils are potential mediators of microvascular injury [40, 41, 45]. This occurrence facilitates increased rolling and sticking of neutrophils onto the endothelial surface (***Figure 1***). In addition to adherence, neutrophil-neutrophil aggregation plays an important role in the occlusion of post-capillary venules during generalized activation, causing tissue ischemia. The result of these phenomena is the formation of a microenvironment between the endothelial cell and the neutrophil. In this microenvironment, neutrophil-derived proteases and toxic oxygen products are present to high relative concentrations and can act synergistically on the endothelial surface, protected from inactivation by circulating plasma antiproteases and free-radical scavengers [46]. This leads to endothelial injury, intercellular gap formation, increased permeability, and neutrophil emigration into the interstitium via diapedesis toward a chemo-attractant gradient. Once in the interstitium, neutrophils come in contact with the extracellular matrix proteins fibronectin and laminin; these proteins upregulate the neutrophil oxidative burst [47]. It should be emphasized that in critically ill patients (including septic patients) a neutrophil dysfunction has been observed (characterized by a markedly depressed chemotaxis, altered intrinsic neutrophil metabolic functions such as production of superoxide and hydrogen peroxide, enzyme content and microbial killing activity [37]. These functional alterations rendered the neutrophils ineffective in defending against invading organisms yet still function as potent inflammatory cells. It therefore appears that - on one hand - suppression of antimicrobial function may increase the vulnerability to infection, while - on the other hand - under the influence of cytokine/mediator "milieu", neutrophils can interact with the endothelial system and macrophages to produce an excessive, uncontrolled systemic inflammation leading to bystander tissue injury and organ dysfunction.

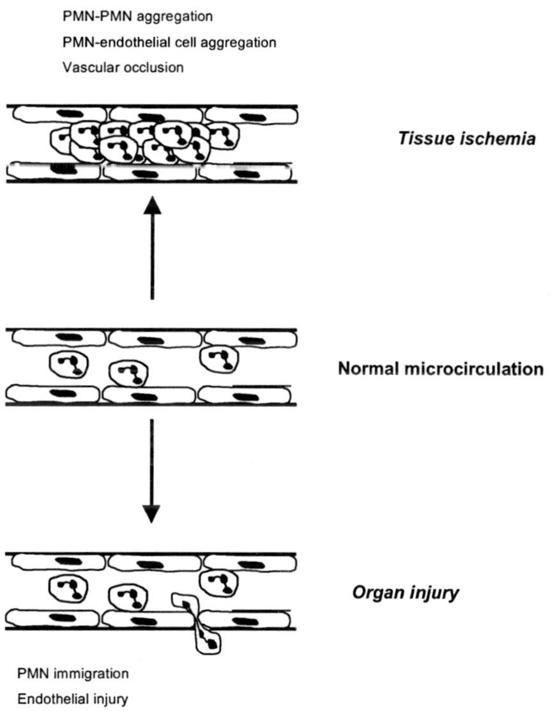

Figure 1. Inflammatory insult causes PMN-PMN aggregation, resulting in microvascular occlusion and tissue ischemia. PMN-endothelial cell aggregation results in microvascular endothelial injury, aggravating tissue damage. PMN immigration into the tissues through the defective endothelium further attenuates tissue/organ injury.

The Role of Microvascular Endothelial Cells

The endothelium is the lining between blood and the tissues. Endothelial cells are in close and intimate contact with blood. In adult humans, the surface area is estimated at > 1000 m^2, roughly the size of a football field [48]. Hence, there is intensive contact of blood cells and plasma proteins with endothelial cells. These cells are not inert cells; indeed, the microvascular endothelium can be viewed as an independent organ. Under physiologic conditions, microvascular endothelial cells exert a number of functions that are important for normal homeostasis [40]. These functions include regulation and / or prevention of coagulation, orchestration of the migration of blood cells into the tissues by expression of adhesion molecules, production of chemo-attractant compounds, regulation of the microcirculation by dictating the tonus of the artelioles, regulation of blood pressure (via their effects on arterioles), and regulation of vasopermeability [49 - 51]. Microvascular endothelial cell injury is the result of endothelial oxidant production, complement activation, platelet aggregation, neutrophil activation, monocyte production of monocytes, arachidonic acid metabolites, and the products of anaerobic metabolism and lactic acidosis [41]. Endothelial cells may adapt their function upon interaction with inflammatory mediators. In addition, they may generate inflammatory mediators themselves. These changes are referred to as "activation of the endothelial cells" or as "malignant intravascular inflammation" [16, 40, 52]. They encompass a change from an anti- into a procoagulant surface (aiming to wall off an infectious process); the expression of adhesion molecules (such as ICAM-1, ELAM-1, vascular cell adhesion molecule-1, P-selectin, E-selectin, etc); the production of inflammatory mediators, including chemo-attractant agents; and the production of vasoactive compounds [49, 53]. Increased microvascular permeability results in edema formation and hypotension form the massive fluid losses into the interstitium. The hypotension and defects in perfusion are exacerbated by the peripheral vasodilatation (decreased systemic vascular resistance) produced by the release of kinins, histamine, and other vasoactive peptides during activation of the inflammatory cascade. The general dysfunction of the endothelium plays a central role in the pathogenesis of sepsis [40]. Of note, not all the endothelial cells display all of these changes. Whether the endothelial cells display all or only some of the features discussed above will depend on the time of stimulation and the nature of the inflammatory stimulus and its concentration. Moreover, the response of the endothelium to inflammatory stimuli may differ greatly at different sites of the body. Together, the interaction among macrophages, neutrophils, and the endothelial system augments the inflammatory cascade and results in bystander organ failure [37]. Microvascular injury is compounded by reperfusion injury in areas made ischemic during the initial stages of sepsis and septic shock.

Cytokines in Sepsis

Macrophage-secreted cytokines are pleomorphic immuno-regulatory peptides acting as potent inflammatory mediators. These molecules mediate the immune / metabolic response to an external stimulus and fuel the transition from sepsis to septic shock, MODS, and / or MOF. Cytokines are a key element in this inflammatory response that characterizes sepsis and septic shock. Synergistic interactions between cytokines can cause or attenuate tissue injury [54]. Therefore, monitoring a profile of cytokines rather than just one cytokine may be necessary.

The most widely investigated cytokines are tumor necrosis factor (TNF), interleukin-1, and interleukin-8, which are generally pro-inflammatory, and interleukin-6 and interleukin-10, which tend to be anti-inflammatory [55]. An infectious or inflammatory trigger, such as a microbial toxin, stimulates the production of TNF and IL-1, which in turn promote endothelial cell-leukocyte adhesion, release of proteases and arachidonate metabolites, and activation of clotting [56 - 59]. Among the mediators produced by the active macrophages TNF is the most important and earliest released [60]. Plasma or serum levels of TNF are elevated in patients with sepsis, although the magnitude of this elevation may depend, in part, on the severity and acuity of the sepsis. TNF injection mimics the pathophysiologic manifestations of sepsis [61]. In addition, TNF can amplify the response to endotoxin by further activating the inflammatory cascade resulting in endothelial damage [62]. The inverse correlation between plasma levels of TNF and survival of patients with meningococcal bacteremia is a strong indicator that TNF has a primary role in the pathogenesis of sepsis [63]. IL-1 and TNF are synergistic and share many biologic effects in sepsis. Their inhibition improves organ function and survival in animal models of sepsis [64, 65]. Experimental studies showed that IL-1 has a role similar to that of TNF in mediating sepsis [66]. They are both involved in the increases in proteolysis and catabolism seen in sepsis and have been implicated in the inflammatory cell response, including endothelial and neutrophil activation. IL-1 induce prostaglandin E_2 synthesis in the anterior hypothalamus resetting the thermoregulatory center to a higher set-point resulting in the symptom of chills and the clinical signs of shivering, rigors, and fever [67]. IL-1 is rarely detected in patients with the sepsis syndrome, but when it is, there is a significant correlation with mortality [68]. In contrast to animal studies, where the infusion of IL-1ra significantly improved survival [69], IL-1ra failed to improve survival in patients with sepsis [70].

Plasma levels of IL-6 (a marker of systemic inflammation) correlated with mortality in patients with sepsis [68]. IL-6 formation is attenuated by the production of either TNF or IL-1. It is possible that IL-6 is toxic only when is produced with other cytokines (synergistic action of cytokines) [54]. IL-8, a neutrophil chemotaxin may have an especially important role in perpetuating tissue inflammation [71, 72]. IL-8 levels correlate with mortality in patients with sepsis [72, 73]. IL-10 functions as an anti-inflammatory cytokine [74]. IL-10 levels relate with the severity of septic shock as measured by the APACHE-II score [75, 76]. IL-2 activates cytotoxic lymphocytes, induces synthesis of other lymphokines, and is a NK- and T-cell growth factor [15]. Obviously, a number of other cytokines are involved in the pathogenesis of sepsis and septic shock and amplify the effects of the above-mentioned inflammatory mediators (synergistic action of cytokines); however, existing data about their precise role are limited at the present time.

Other Inflammatory Mediators

Reactive Oxygen Species

Reactive oxygen species are produced by leukocytes as part of the normal host defense against infecting microorganisms. Reactive oxygen species disorganize cell membranes and lead to cell necrosis. Changes after injury, ischemia / reperfusion, or both my lead to excessive production of these harmful molecules with deleterious effects on organ function (**Figure 2**) [77].

Nitric Oxide ($NO^{\cdot}$)

Excessive $NO^{\cdot}$ production is involved in the pathogenesis of sepsis and sepsis syndrome and MODS and is one of the many effector molecules in the complex cytokine/hormonal network in patients with sepsis [78, 79].

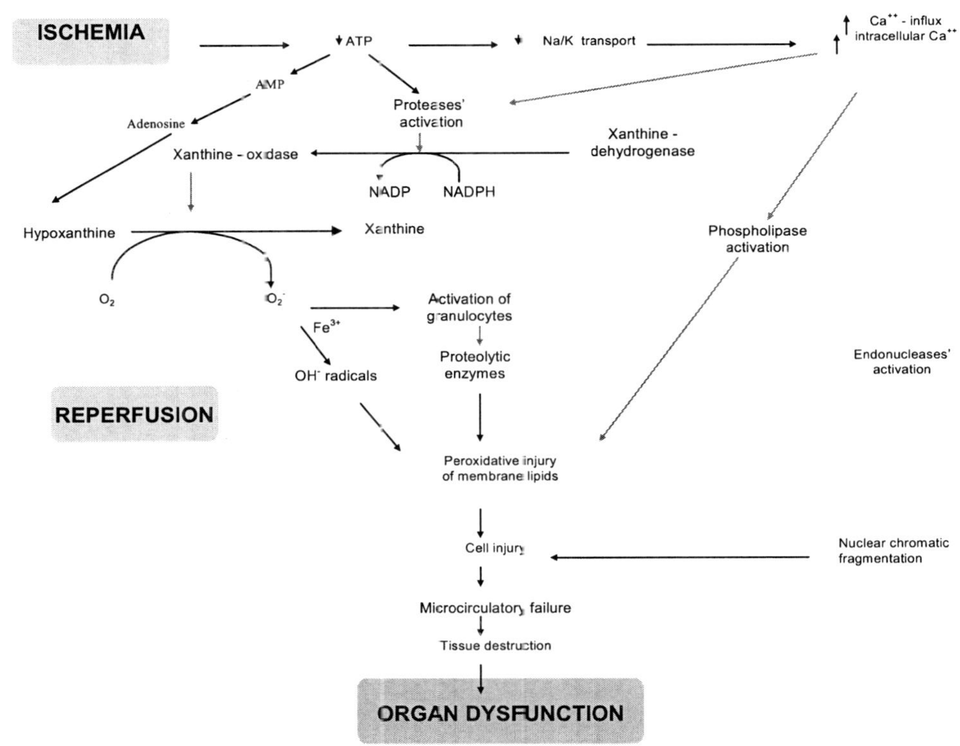

Figure 2 (legend). Pathophysiology of ischemia / reperfusion organ injury. Oxygen free radicals, activation of polymorphonuclear leukocytes (PMN), failure of microvascular perfusion, cellular acidosis, a disturbance of cytosolic free calcium, and inflammatory mediators are among the underlying pathogenetic mechanisms in the pathophysiology of ischemia / reperfusion tissue / organ injury. For a detailed discussion about the pathophysiology of ischemia / reperfusion - induced organ injury, see ref. No 77.

Phospholipase A_2. (PLA_2)

PLA_2 contributes to the inflammatory response by the production of arachidonic acid (leading to the release of eicosanoids) and by the formation of PAF [80, 81]. Both of these end products are potent mediators of the inflammatory cascade [80, 81].

Platelet Activating Factor (PAF)

PAF is produced by a host of inflammatory cell types, including neutrophils, macrophages, platelets, endothelial cells, and fibroblasts. PAF is a PLA_2 – dependent, potent, effector pro-inflammatory agent capable of eliciting platelet aggregation, neutrophil aggregation and degranulation, and changes in vascular smooth-muscle tone by binding to cell-surface receptors and by participating in complex intracellular and intercellular signaling systems [82, 83]. PAF – like some of the prostaglandins – acts as a secondary mediator of some of the functions of the major cytokines [67]. This biological action results in microvascular injury.

Eicosanoids

Eicosanoids are the metabolic products of arachidonic acid. The enzyme cyclooxygenase catalyzes the synthesis of prostaglandins and thromboxane A_2, and lipo-oxyzenase converts arachidonic acid to leukotrienes [84]. Eicosanoids are known to have powerful effects on host tissue and inflammatory cells and induce profound vasoconstriction, platelet aggregation, neutrophil infiltration, and increased vascular permeability [84, 85].

Coagulation Disorders in Sepsis

Severe sepsis is almost invariably associated with activation of the coagulation system [86, 87]. As previously noted, cytokines cause endothelial cells to loose their anti-thrombotic state, up-regulate the expression of leukocyte adhesion molecules, and synthesize chemotactic cytokines [88]. TNF and IL-1 induce endothelial cell expression of tissue factor, decrease the activity of the thrombomodulin-protein C anticoagulation pathway, decrease production of tissue-type plasminogen activator, and increase production of plasminogen activator inhibitor [88]. The net effect is to promote fibrin deposition and the microaggregation of microthrombi composed of platelets, PMNLs, RBCs, and fibrin, which may obstruct the small capillaries and impair the delivery of blood and substrate to the tissues (tissue ischemia) [89].

The severity of the derangement of coagulation may range from mere laboratory abnormalities without much clinical relevance to widespread and systemic deposition of fibrin (leading to impaired organ perfusion and contributing to organ dysfunction) and simultaneous consumption of coagulation factors and platelets, potentially resulting in bleeding [90]. Most clinicians recognize this syndrome as disseminated intravascular coagulation (DIC) [88 - 90]. In the pathogenesis of severe coagulation abnormalities in sepsis, three major mechanisms appear to play a role: (a) tissue factor-driven generation of thrombin and subsequent fibrinogen to fibrin conversion and platelet activation (b) impairment of all major physiologic anticoagulant mechanisms, that is, the anti-thrombin system, the protein C system, and the tissue factor pathway inhibitor (TFPI) system; and (c) a plasminogen activator inhibitor type1-mediated shutdown of the fibrinolytic system [89, 90].

In addition to these coagulation disorders observed in sepsis, there is evidence that there are defective red blood cells with altered shapes or rheologic properties that may predispose to plugging or obstruction of the microvasculature and result in cellular or tissue ischemia [91]. In the presence of the activated coagulation system and endothelial abnormalities characteristic of the inflammatory state, these altered red blood cells may further contribute to the perfusion abnormalities that may result in MODS/MOF [54, 86].

Complement Activation

Inappropriate or excessive activation of the complement system can lead to harmful, potentially life-threatening consequences due to severe inflammatory tissue destruction. Activation of the complement cascade can occur by either the usual or alternate pathways and – when activated systemically – contributes to increased vascular permeability, endothelial cell damage, and release of secondary mediators, such as leukotrienes, prostaglandins, histamine and other compounds released by degranulating mast cells, and PAF [67]. These consequences are clinically manifested in various disorders, including septic shock and MODS / MOF [92]. The C5a fragment of the complement is implicated as a particularly potent mediator of the inflammatory process [41]. Genetic complement deficiencies or complement depletion have been proven to be beneficial in reducing tissue injury in a number of animal models of severe complement-dependent inflammation. It is therefore believed that therapeutic inhibition of complement (for example, by antibodies directed against C5a) is likely to arrest the process of certain diseases, including septic shock and sepsis-induced MODS / MOF [93].

The Role of the Gastrointestinal Tract

The gastrointestinal tract epithelium plays an important role in the development of MODS/MOF in septic patients. Following hemorrhagic shock, septic shock, or LPS infusion, an alteration in the function of the intestinal epithelium as a barrier between the enteric flora and the portal circulation has been repeatedly shown [94 - 97]. This abnormal cell function relates to mucosal cell injury or death. The terminal ileum and cecum are large reservoirs for gram-negative bacteria and their toxic products, such as endotoxin. Bacterial overgrowth commonly occurs in critically ill septic patients. Bacterial overgrowth, intestinal mucosa damage, and altered host immune functions result in a failure of gut antibacterial defenses [95]. Because of the increased intestinal mucosal permeability, these bacteria and/or their toxic products may translocate through or between the dysfunctional intestinal mucosal barrier cells and enter the mesenteric lymph system (endogenous endotoxemia and bacterial translocation) [94, 95]. If they are not adequately neutralized by the mesenteric lymph nodes, they may enter the systemic circulation or the portal circulation, causing an ongoing stimulation of the immuno-inflammatory defense system, an attenuation of the injury state, and potentially MODS and/or MOF (***Figure 3***) [96, 97]. The susceptibility of the splanchnic circulation to reduction to flow as a response to shock, the relatively high concentration of xanthine oxidase in the gastrointestinal mucosa and microvascular endothelium, and the presence of endogenous flora support this theory [94].

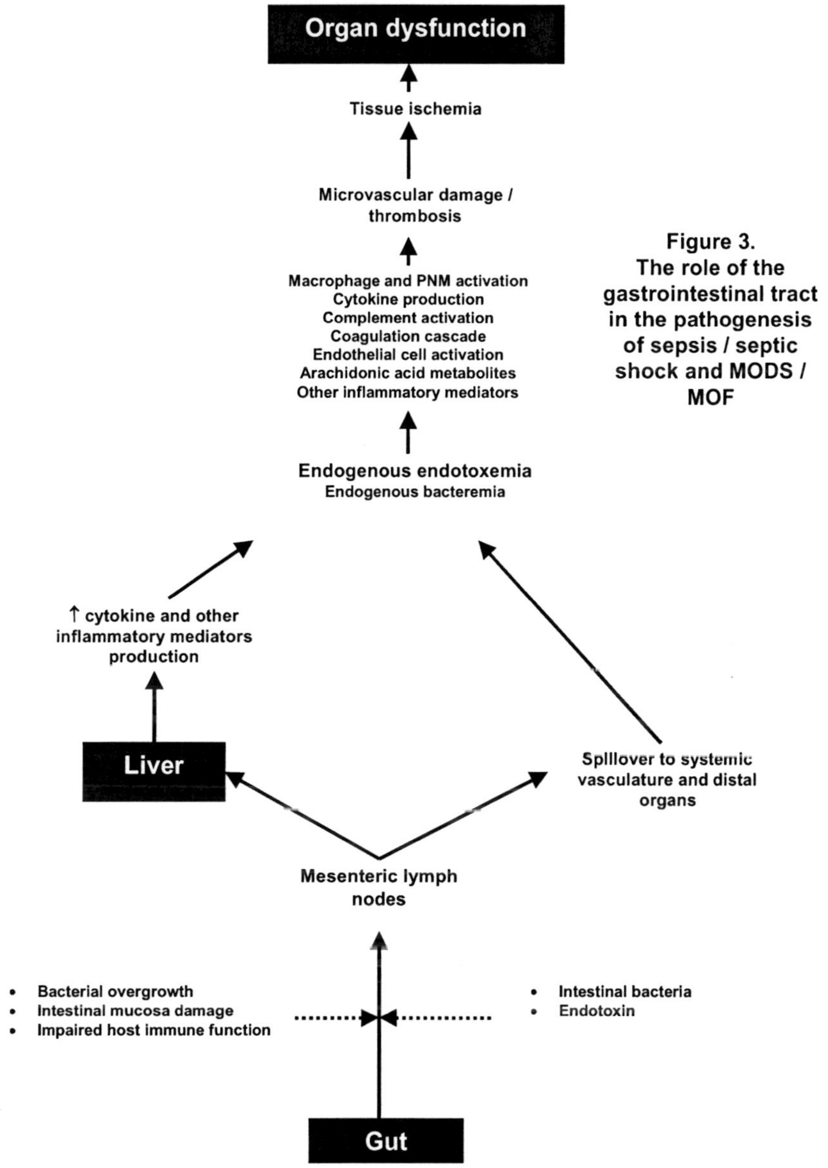

Figure 3. The role of the gastrointestinal tract in the pathogenesis of sepsis / septic shock and MODS / MOF

The Role of the Liver

The liver is a key organ in sepsis. The liver receives about 25 % of total cardiac output, mainly from the splanchnicomesenteric vascular bed, a region especially subject to vasoconstriction and bacterial translocation during sepsis. The cellular population of the liver (including hepatocytes, Kuppfer cells, and endothelial sinusoidal cells) is actively involved in the immune, anti-infectious, and metabolic responses through multiple cell cross talk and interactions [98]. Hepatic inflammatory and coagulation processes in sepsis may alter the function of this organ. Indeed, the liver can by injured by activated Kuppfer cells that release chemokines, attract blood neutrophils into the liver, and activate them. Neutrophils upregulate their surface adhesion molecules and bind to sinusoidal cells. Upregulation of endothelial integrins promotes neutrophil migration and microvascular thrombi. After migrating into the parenchyma, activated neutrophils produce oxygen-derived radicals and proteases that may injury hepatocytes. This cascade may lead to microcirculatory disturbances, fibrin deposition, hepatocyte injury, endotoxin and bacteria spillover, enhanced inflammatory processes, and multiple organ failure [98]. Additional injury to both endothelial cells and associated parenchymal cells occurs with the initiation of resuscitation. A number of mediators of reperfusion injury are produced and released and contribute to enhanced tissue injury [99].

Myocardial Depression in Septic Shock

Myocardial depression, like vascular dysfunction, is typical in septic shock. The decreased cardiac filling and cardiac output may be exacerbated by the direct myocardial depression associated with sepsis. Human septic myocardial depression is characterized by reversible biventricular dilatation, increased end-diastolic volume, decreased ejection fraction, and decreased response to fluid resuscitation and catecholamine stimulation, even though the stroke volume and the cardiac output may be adequately maintained or even increased (i.e., even in the presence of overall hyperdynamic circulation) [16, 100, 101]. A circulating myocardial depressant factor, not myocardial hypoperfusion, is responsible for this phenomenon [102]. This substance has been shown to represent low concentrations of TNF-α and IL-1β acting in synergy on the myocardium through mechanisms that include NO and cGMP generation [101].

Apoptosis in Septic Shock

Apoptosis is the programmed cell death; it is characterized by nuclear degeneration, condensation, nuclear DNA degradation, and phagocytosis of cell residua. There is evidence that increased apoptotic processes may play a significant role in the outcome to sepsis syndromes [103]. In particular, increased apoptosis, especially in lymphoid tissues and potentially in some parenchymal tissues from solid organs may contribute to immune suppression secondary to apoptotic losses in T cell, B cell, and NK cell populations. These alterations may contribute significantly to the risk of secondary opportunistic infections and to the risk of development of complications of sepsis, such as MODS and even MOF [103].

Neuroendocrine Reflex

Septic shock, with its associated reduction in functional blood volume, hypotension, and tissue damage, leads to the known neuroendocrine response to stress [104, 105]. This neuroendocrine reflex during the early phases of septic shock is designed to maintain cardiac and cerebral perfusion via peripheral vasoconstriction and reflex tachycardia. These effects are mediated through the sympathetic nervous system and adrenal medullary release of catecholamines as part of the stress syndrome. As the selective redistribution of flow occurs, reduction in renal flow and adrenal flow eventually results in activation of the renin-angiotensin system and adrenocortical hormone release. Further loss of intravascular volume results in a drop in cardiac output and a reduction in blood flow to different organs. With further volume shifts, cardiac and cerebral perfusion is maintained by selective reduction in flow to the renal and splanchnic beds, resulting in oliguria and mesenteric ischemia. Beyond this point, further reduction in volume exceeds the compensatory mechanisms, hypotension ensues (mean arterial pressure [MAP] < 70 mm Hg) and adequate cerebral and coronary perfusion can no longer be maintained [104, 105]. This is manifested as anxiety and combativeness, then lethargy, and finally loss of consciousness [41].

Critical Illness Polyneuropathy

The development of neuromuscular weakness recently has been recognized as a potential complication in this group of patients and has been termed critical illness polyneuropathy or polymyopathy [106]. In the pathogenesis of this syndrome, a primary axonal degeneration (likely resulting from proinflammatory mediators) is involved. Sufficient axons' recover may be achieved even after 3 – 6 months [106]. Critical illness polyneuropathy may explain prolonged ventilatory dependency in some critically ill patients and may necessitate rehabilitation efforts even after weaning or separation from ventilatory support before the patients are able to return home and care for themselves.

Genetic Predisposition to Sepsis and Septic Shock

Genotype has been shown to contribute substantially to outcome in inflammatory and infectious diseases [107 - 109]. The severity of sepsis differs among patients. It is possible that genetic factors may have important roles in the evolution of and final outcome from infection, sepsis syndrome, and septic shock [108, 110]. The possibility of gene polymorphism that could either protect against septic shock or increase sensitivity to bacterial infections is currently under intense investigation. In depth understanding of the pathophysiology of sepsis and the role of genetic factors may eventually translate into effective individualized preventive and treatment strategies in the future.

Other Causes of Organ / System Dusfunction in Septic Shock

In some septic patients, the underlying disease process or some of the therapeutic schemas may be responsible for the organ or system dysfunction. A typical example is the renal dysfunction following the therapeutic administration of aminoglycosides or other nephrotoxic agents (such as amphotericin, contrast materials etc). All the potentially undesirable adverse effects of therapeutic agents and / or diagnostic procedures (i.e. intravenous administration of a contrast agent) should be considered in the septic patient with organ dysfunction and – when possible – the potentially offending agents must be stopped or changed to avoid the deterioration of organ function and the development of organ failure [2, 3, 16, 41].

Metabolic Derangements in Sepsis and Septic Shock

Metabolic derangements are frequently observed among septic patients. These patients may be particularly at risk for the development of severe malnutrition [111]. This complication may compromise the patient's immune function and the ability to mount an adequate inflammatory response against the offending organism. Cellular energy charge is usually maintained in the early stages of sepsis. Worsening or late sepsis is characterized by a decrease in cellular energy charge secondary to mal-distribution of blood flow (which contains oxygen and nutrients) and inadequate oxygen delivery and tissue hypoxia, resulting in anaerobic glycolysis and lactic acid production [52, 91, 112]. The decline in energy production results from sepsis-induced mitochondrial dysfunction, a process that has been termed "cytopathic hypoxia" [112, 113]. The period of ischemia may be followed by reperfusion and oxidative injury, which may produce organ system dysfunction / failure [77, 91]. The metabolic changes associated with sepsis are summarized in ***Table 6*** [112].

Table 6. Metabolic alterations in sepsis

Carbohydratc metabolism	Lipid Metabolism	Protein metabolism
Whole body uptake of glucose ↑	Lipolytic activity ↑	Protein catabolism ↑ (especially in skeletal muscle, gut and connective tissue)
Glycolysis ↑	Hypertriglyceridemia	Synthesis of acute phase proteins ↑ (in late phases of sepsis ↓)
Insulin resistance ↑	Fatty infiltration of the liver ↑	Synthesis of visceral proteins of homeostasis (e.g., albumin) ↓
Glyconeogenesis (from lactate, the Cori cycle) ↑ Hyperlactatemia Metabolic acidosis	Ketogenesis ↓	

Microbiologic Considerations in Septic Shock

In severe sepsis, clinical outcome depends on microbiologic factors. During the 1950s to the early 1980s, sepsis was primarily attributable to gram-negative organisms [114]. Even though the incidence of sepsis with gram-negative organisms appears to be decreasing from its levels of the 1970s and 1980s, it continues to be frequently encountered, and gram-negative organisms are a major cause of nosocomial infections [26]. Nowadays, gram-positive organisms are responsible for approximately 50 % of bacteremic events [32, 115]. Gram-positive microorganisms can trigger sepsis and septic shock by the production and release of exotoxins acting as "super-antigens" and by the release of cell membrane fragments (including peptidoglycans, teichoic acids, and lipoteichoic acids) that can trigger the inflammatory cascade (see above) [116, 117]. Mortality caused by gram-positive bacteremia has equaled or exceeded death caused by gram-negative bacteremia [1, 118]. The National Nosocomial Infections Surveillance (NNIS) system reported that between 1992 and 1997 coagulase-negative staphylococci were the most common blood stream isolates [26]. Enterococci and Staphylococcus aureus were the next most commonly isolated organisms in the blood. The lung is the most common site of infection, followed by the abdomen and urinary tract [3]. The source of infection seems to be an important determinant of clinical outcome. The greatest risk of developing severe sepsis occurs in the setting of bacteremia associated with nosocomial pneumonia [119]. Patients with intraabdominal infections and polymicrobial bacteremia or postoperative wound infections and bacteremia are at significant risk for severe sepsis [119]. Bacteremia associated with intravascular catheters or indwelling urinary catheters carries a lower risk of developing septic shock [115]. Nosocomial pneumonia and urinary tract infections are most frequently attributable to gram-negative bacteria. S. Aureus also was a frequent cause of hospital-acquired pneumonia [26]. Various pathogens have been identified that increase the risk for shock and death. Bloodstream infection caused by Pseudomonas aeruginosa, Candida albicans, or multi-drug resistant Enterococcus faecium is associated with increased mortality [120 - 122].

In 20 – 30 % of patients, and despite intensive diagnostic investigation with the aid of highly sophisticated diagnostic tools (including computed tomography), a definite site of infection is not determined [33]. Small infections in the pleural and / or peritoneal space and in paranasal-sinus infections can easily be overlooked. It should be emphasized that bloodstream invasion is not necessary for the development of septic shock; indeed, only 30 – 50 % of patients with sepsis have positive blood culture results [3, 33]. Of note, the clinical picture of septic shock may be caused by inflammatory disorders not caused by infection (such as severe acute pancreatitis); these patients have biochemical and physiologic changes, rates of organ failure, and survival rates similar to those of patients with confirmed infection [30]. Diagnostic aspiration (CT- or US-guided, if necessary) should be performed to obtain material for culture; antibiotherapy should be based on the results of culture [123]. Diagnostic approach and therapeutic management of the septic patient will be discussed (see below).

Chapter 4

Diagnostic Evaluation of the Septic Patient

Early recognition of sepsis is of key importance for successful treatment. During the diagnostic evaluation of the septic patient, the goals of the clinician are the following:

- The identification of sepsis as the cause of the clinical picture
- The localization of the site of infection, and
- The interpretation of the microbiologic findings

The differential diagnosis between sepsis and non-infective systemic inflammatory response syndrome (SIRS) may be particularly difficult. An important first step is a systemic consideration of all possible non-infectious causes of SIRS (***Table 7***).

Fever is a common sign in hospitalized patients and may be due to infectious and non-infectious causes [124] (***Table 8***). On the other hand, there are some patients with sepsis - for example, elderly patients or patients with uremia – in whom fever is not observed [125]. The lack of a febrile reaction indicates the absence of an acute-phase response and it usually reflects the immunosuppressive phase of sepsis; this clinical picture is associated with an obscure prognosis and a high mortality. Subtle changes in the mental status represent a particularly useful early manifestation of sepsis and should be viewed with a high index of suspicion for the presence of severe sepsis.

Table 7. Non-infectious causes of SIRS

Tissue injury
Surgery / Trauma
Hematoma / Venous thrombosis
Myocardial / Pulmonary infarction
Transplant rejection
Pancreatitis
Erythroderma
Metabolic
Thyroid storm
Acute adrenal insufficiency
Therapy related
Blood products
Cytokines, especially granulocyte-macrophage colony stimulating factor (GM-CSF)
Anesthetic-related malignant hyperpyrexia, especially halothane
Neuroleptic malignant syndrome, for example caused by haloperidol
Opiates / benzodiazepines
Malignancy
Hypernephroma / lymphoma
Tumor lysis syndrome
Neurological
Subarachnoid hemorrhage

To detect the potential sources of sepsis and to guide subsequent investigation and management, focused clinical examination, guided by the recognition of risk factors relevant to the individual patient, should be the next step. Surgical and traumatic wounds should be exposed and examined for signs of infection. Particular attention should be paid to vascular access sites for signs of phlebitis or cellulites and to pressure areas or injection sites for evidence of soft tissue infection. Evidence of sinusitis should be sought, and fundoscopy is invaluable in detecting candidal endophthalmitis, a pathognomonic feature of systemic fungal sepsis. Urinalysis may indicate urinary tract infection; in severe cases, urine in the catheter may be frankly purulent. The presence of diarrhea may indicate *Clostridium Difficile* associated colitis [126]. Repeated, complete physical examination is invaluable in order to detect the emergence of new signs. However, the localization of the site of infection may be difficult and confounded by the fact that there are multiple pathological processes occurring concurrently in the critically ill patient.

Table 8. Infectious and non-infectious causes of fever in the ICU

Infected intravascular catheters
Sinusitis or otitis media (in patients with intranasal devices such as nasogastric tubes or nasal endotracheal tubes)
Acalculous cholecystitis
Drug fever
Pulmonary emboli
Deep venous thrombosis
Central fever (in patients with head trauma)
Clostridium Difficile colitis
Postcardiotomy syndrome
Secondary infection by resistant organisms
Fungal infection

The interpretation of microbiological findings is frequently difficult in septic patients for a variety of reasons:

- Frequent use of antibiotic therapy
- Need to differentiate colonization from infection
- Correct identification of unfamiliar microorganism may be difficult
- Need to determine the significance of mixed culture results
- Need to estimate the clinical importance of microorganisms normally of low virulence

Principal among these factors is that many organisms isolated from non-sterile sites may represent either colonization or infection – microbiology alone cannot answer this question. Conversely, the microbiology laboratory may report negative results in samples that are in fact infected, either because antibiotics have sterilized the specimen, or because special procedures need to be carried out (for example, immuno-fluorescence to detect *Pneumocystis carinii*).

An increase or decrease in white-cell count or an increase in the immature to total neutrophil ratio is an early manifestation of sepsis. However, neutrophilia lacks sufficient sensitivity among hospitalized patients to be of value in distinguishing sepsis, although marked neutrophilia or failure to mount a neutrophil response may be of prognostic value [126]. An elevated blood-glucose level is another early manifestation of sepsis. Levels of procalcitonin (PCT) and C-reactive protein (CRP) are straightforward to assay. These acute-phase markers may be useful in the differential diagnosis of infection from other causes of SIRS [127]. Levels of CRP and PCT are correlated with the degree of inflammatory response and are of particular value in monitoring response to treatment [128]. PCT may have some advantages over CRP in that it rises more quickly at the onset of inflammation and is cleared more quickly as inflammation resolves [129]. Levels of PCT are correlated more closely with severity of sepsis [130] and also are predictive of mortality [131]. A prospective study of ICU patients found that a CRP level of 50 mg/l or higher had a sensitivity of 98.5 % and specificity of 75 % in identifying probable or definite sepsis [132]. De Werra et al [133], also in an ICU population, found PCT levels of 1.5 ng/ml or higher to have a sensitivity of 100 % and specificity of 72 % in identifying sepsis. In a prospective study of 175 children admitted to a PICU, Hatherill et al [134] found that procalcitonin levels were more useful in identifying the presence of bacterial infection than was C-reactive protein, which was more useful than was the leukocyte count. These serologic markers should be used as a part of a systemic evaluation that includes clinical examination and different diagnostic techniques. Daily, sequential measurement of inflammatory markers is likely to be of more value in diagnosis of infection than single measurements [133].

Detection of circulating endotoxin is another potentially specific test for sepsis. These measurements, however, are associated with many problems (such as wide variation of the sensitivity, lack of defined cutoffs, and the transient nature of endotoxemia), and - for these reasons - measurements of endotoxin levels in septic patients remains experimental.

Chapter 5

Management of Septic Shock

The initial management of patients with septic shock is predominantly supportive. Early recognition of the syndrome is of crucial importance to start promptly the appropriate management. Timely, aggressive resuscitation to preserve organ function remains a fundamental principle in the care of septic patients [135]. Effective organ support is essential because it is the cumulative burden of organ failure that leads to death [135, 136]. The specific treatment is directed at identifying and treating the underlying disorder. The patient should be investigated diligently in an effort to identify an active infection; modern imaging techniques are invaluable in the diagnostic evaluation of the septic patient. Every attempt should be made to obtain adequate culture specimens from potential infective sources [16] (see below]. Early administration of appropriate, effective antibiotic therapy and – when indicated – aggressive and effectual drainage (of infected fluid collections) or surgical debridement (of infected necrotic tissues), without delay, is two therapeutic interventions especially important in the management of septic patients [137].

Supportive Therapy

Immediate resuscitation and stabilization of the respiratory and cardiovascular systems are the first management considerations in the patient with septic shock, as in shock of other etiologies [137, 138]. However, supportive therapy is not a therapeutic option for the management of septic patients, and thus the goal is to support the individual failing organ/system until the indications requiring supportive therapy are reversed.

Pulmonary Dysfunction

In the septic patient, many alterations in the pulmonary function have been observed, including significant disturbances of gas exchange (caused by an extensive right-to-left intrapulmonary shunting of blood flow), decreased lung compliance, increased airway resistance related to small airway and alveolar collapse, increased work of breathing, and impairment of muscle efficiency [139, 140]. Control of the upper airway and consideration of the need for ventilatory support is an important first step in the management of the patients with respiratory dysfunction related to sepsis. High minute ventilation is required; oxygen should be administered immediately by mask, provided that the airway is patent and the patient is breathing adequately. Arterial blood gases should be measured; arterial oxyhemoglobin saturation should be maintained above 90 %. If the patient cannot adequately protect his/her airway or if respirations appear to be ineffective, an endotracheal tube should be placed immediately; in this case, mechanical ventilation is indicated [138]. Commonly accepted indications for institution of mechanical ventilation from other causes or respiratory failure apply equally to septic patients, including refractory hypoxemia ($P_aO_2 < 60$ despite high flow oxygen), respiratory rate more than 35 breaths / min, and vital capacity below 15 ml/kg, among others [140]. Because of increased rates of sinusitis, orotracheal intubation is the preferred route [140]. One of the chief benefits of mechanical ventilatory support is to reduce patient's work of breathing so that blood flow may be redirected to other vital organs.

There is no strong evidence that one ventilatory strategy is superior to others [141, 142]. Volume-cycled ventilation using the "assist-control" mode (controlled mandatory ventilation) is an appropriate mode to choose at the outset [140]. Similar degrees of respiratory support can probably be achieved with intermitted mandatory ventilation or pressure-regulated volume-controlled ventilation [140]. When PEEP is used, usually low PEEP levels (5 – 10 cm H_2O) are used initially until oxygen requirements exceed 40 to 60 %; after this point, PEEP is increased [143]. Although the highest safe level of supplemental oxygen is uncertain, the potential risk of oxygen toxicity should not supersede the immediate risk of hypoxia. A balanced use of PEEP and supplemental oxygen can achieve an arterial saturation of 90 % (an approximate pO_2 of 60 mm Hg). Tidal volume should be chosen based on ideal body weight and should be targeted to prevent end-inspiratory plateau pressures from exceeding 30 cm H_2O whenever possible [140]. Permissive hypercapnia (the method of allowing CO_2 to rise while reducing tidal volume and minute ventilation to prevent alveolar over-distension or propagation of lung injury) has been proven to be effective in reducing mortality without adverse consequences [144].

Nearly 85 % of patients with septic shock require ventilatory support, typically for 7 – 14 days [3]. Interestingly, although functional impairment can take months to resolve and sub-clinical spirometric changes are sometimes permanent, unremitting lung failure is uncommon [145]. Since intubation and mechanical ventilation are associated with significant ongoing risk, every attempt should be made to discontinue mechanical ventilation as rapidly as is safely possible [146]. This effort is made as usually (i.e., by reducing toxic F_{IO2} and using the least toxic F_{IO2} consistent with adequate arterial saturation, lowering PEEP, and progressively liberating the patient from mechanical ventilation).

Cardiovascular Dysfunction

In the septic patient, it is important to restore and maintain hemodynamic stability [16, 135]. Clinical parameters, such as mentation, heart rate, blood pressure, urine output, and skin perfusion, provide useful, but limited information regarding cardiovascular performance [3, 34, 37, 135, 147]. Invasive monitoring with pulmonary artery catheterization guides the implementation of effective care and is indicated especially in patients with myocardial, pulmonary, of renal dysfunction; despite some controversy [148, 149], early invasive monitoring has been associated with improved resuscitative parameters and survival [150]. Cardiovascular management aims to maintain a cardiac output and oxygen delivery adequate to reverse tissue hypoperfusion; however, adverse effects of excessive therapy should be avoided. The initial agent should be fluid to ensure that the circulating intravascular volume is appropriate and that tissue perfusion is restored and cellular metabolism is normalized [151]. Fluid resuscitation should commence with infusion of crystalloid solutions. The amount of fluid required varies greatly among patients and stages of their disease. Many patients will require 4 – 6 lt of crystalloid-containing fluid [152]. Fluid administration is guided by the response to therapy. Despite some continuing controversy regarding the use of crystalloid versus colloid solutions [153, 154], colloid has no proven advantage over crystalloid [152 - 155].

Hypotension persisting after volume repletion is frequently the result of low systemic vascular resistance occasionally combined with a reduced cardiac index.

In these instances, septic patients require adrenergic therapy in addition to fluid resuscitation to improve tissue / organ perfusion. Alpha-adrenergic agonists are drugs that can boost systemic vascular resistance [156]. Adrenergic support improve outcome from septic shock [151]. All these drugs, except phenylephrine, have marked beta-adrenergic properties as well, increasing the heart rate and myocardial contractility. Dopamine is often used first because it also stimulates dopaminergic receptors, potentially increasing renal blood flow. Initiation of vasopressor therapy should begin at low doses and be titrated to effect ***(Table 9)*** [157]. In patients with severe hypotension, in spite of aggressive fluid and dopamine, dobutamine therapies, or both, alpha-agonists such as norepinephrine (0,01 – 0,1 μgr / kgr / min) or epinephrine (0,01 to 0,1 μgr / kgr / min) have been

Table 9. Vasoactive drug therapy in the patient with septic shock

Awaiting adequate volume repletion, institute multipurpose agent (dopamine or epinephrine) and increase dose from 1 toward 10 (μg/kg/min for dopamine, mg/min for epinephrine) as needed to maintain blood pressure If higher doses are needed, add norepinephrine (2 - 20 μg/min) Discontinue these drugs as urgently as volume repletion and hemostasis allow	Avoid vasoactive drugs until heart "too full" Except dopamine (2 – 5 μg/kg/min) for renal perfusion early Nitroglycerin and nitroprusside are contraindicated Vasoconstictors delay adequate volume repletion If right heart overload with shock, norepinephrine (2 – 20 μg/min) may help by maintaining RV perfusion; in septic shock, vasoconstrictors may help when adequate volume replacement provides inadequate perfusion pressure	Dobutamine (5 – 15 μg/kg/min) to enhance contractility without excess tachycardia, arrhythmia, or vasoconstriction; higher doses dilate skeletal vascular bed Dopamine (2 – 5 μg/kg/min) to preserve renal cortical blood flow; at higher dose (4 – 12 μg/kg/min), increases heart rate, contractility, venous tone, and preload, like epinephrine. Nitroglycerine (25 – 250 μg/min) for venodilation with minimal arterial dilation except for the coronary circulation Sodium nitroprusside (0.1 – 5 μg/kg/min) for arterial dilation to reduce after load and allow greater ejection from a depressed left ventricle or regurgitant aortic/mitral valve

From Ref # 157

used as a temporizing measure [41]. It should be noted that the use of inotropic and vasoactive agents may be associated with the development of arrhytmias and even ischemia of some selected organ beds, such as splanchnic and renal circulatory beds, culminating in ischemic bowel and acute tubular necrosis, respectively [158].

Increased production of lactic acid is the result of global or regional ischemia. Lactic acidosis should be managed by treating the underlying disorder. The administration of bicarbonate is not beneficial regarding the cardiovascular performance, and should be reserved when pH is below 7.2 [159]. Manipulations aiming to increase oxygen delivery / oxygen carrying capacity of the blood (i.e., red blood cell transfusion) [160, 161] have no demonstrated benefit in the management of patients with septic shock [162]. The optimal hemoglobin and hematocrit for patients with septic shock is uncertain. Most experts recommend hemoglobin levels of 9 – 10 g/dl in patients with septic shock [163]. This degree of anemia is usually well tolerated in most patients, even with cardiac impairment [151]. It should be remembered that blood transfusions may be associated with transmission of infectious agents, immune suppression, microcirculatory dysfunction, and even a reduced survival rate [162, 163]. When considering blood transfusion to improve oxygenation in septic patients, stored blood may be less effective than fresh blood [165].

Renal Dysfunction

Hypotension and oliguria in septic patients are initially treated with rapid intravenous fluid administration [67]. Crystalloids are the best fluids to begin with because they are usually immediately available and can be infused rapidly. Repeated infusion of 0.5 lt boluses of fluid, each over 5 - 15 min, is given until the blood pressure and urine output increase to an acceptable level or until signs of pulmonary congestion and elevated jugular venous pressure supervene. Patients poorly responsible to acute volume expansion or patients with severe myocardial or pulmonary dysfunction will usually require aggressive hemodynamic monitoring [150]. Obviously, if urinary flow ceases abruptly, obstructive uropathy must be ruled out. Oliguria in the presence of clinically adequate hemodynamics should prompt examination of the urinary electrolytes to help distinguish acute renal failure from prerenal oliguria and consideration of other possible causes of renal insufficiency (obstruction, primary renal disease). Dialysis is required in fewer than 5 % of patients with renal dysfunction, and eventually recovery is common [166].

General Supportive Measures

General supportive measures include prompt and appropriate nutritional support (see below), prevention of nosocomial infections, stress ulcers (by the administration of histamine antagonists, proton-pump inhibitors, or sucralfate), skin breakdown, deep venous thrombosis (by the administration of low-molecular-weight heparin, and use of venous-compression devices), and judicious use of sedation [167 - 169]. These measures are always beneficial and should be used in the management of the septic patient [135].

Antibiotic Therapy

Microbiological diagnosis aims to identify the responsible microorganism. Its importance is due to many reasons [126, 170]:

i. To make sure that effective antimicrobial therapy is given.
ii. To establish and update a local epidemiologic database at a given hospital regarding prevalence of microorganisms and antimicrobial resistance patterns; these data are essential and should be taken into consideration when empirical therapy is planned.
iii. To determine the indication for adjunctive therapy. At present, this is still an experimental method; however, in the future it may become a useful therapeutic method (see below).

It should be emphasized that antibiotics administration is essential, but not sufficient for the optimal and radical treatment of septic patients. Localization and surgical removal of the nidus of infection remains the most important step in the management of patients with sepsis [3, 16, 37, 135, 147, 171] (see below, "Source control"). However, rapid initiation of adequate and appropriate antibiotic therapy has been shown to improve outcome [114, 119]; despite that, mortality remains significant. It has been estimated that about 10 % of patients do not receive appropriate antibiotic therapy, and the mortality rate is 10 – 15 % higher for such patients than for those who are covered by the appropriate antibiotic therapy [172]. Antibiotic selection is usually empiric and should be based on a combination of factors, including the suspected source / site of infection, the most likely pathogens, the acquisition of the organism from the community or hospital, the knowledge of antibiotic susceptibility patterns for community- and hospital-acquired infections, and on specific host factors (such as the presence and the degree of immune deficiency). A common approach is to initiate broad antibiotic coverage when the pathogen is uncertain; as the results of microbiologic studies become available, antibiotic therapy should be modified to an agent with specific narrow spectrum of activity. Potential side effects (i.e., nephrotoxicity of aminoglycosides, hypersensitivity to β-lactams etc) should be taken into consideration, especially for the critically ill patient in whom organ dysfunction is already present. Dosing requirements should be individualized, especially when the drugs have high potential toxicities (e.g., aminoglycosides). The duration of therapy should be dictated by the clinical response and the laboratory findings (fever, leukocytosis, and presence and degree of granulocytosis) [173]. Unfortunately, indiscriminate use of broad-spectrum antibiotics has led to the development of resistant strains. The emergence of resistance among a variety of microorganisms may limit antibiotic selection for hospital-acquired infections [174, 175]. Enterococci and pneumococci, organisms, once susceptible to many commonly used antibiotics, have developed widespread resistance [174]. Among community-acquired infections, the incidence of penicillin-resistant Streptococcus pneumoniae is increasing [176]. Methicillin-resistant S. aureus is a major problem in many hospitals, mandating the addition of intravenous vancomycin in most cases of septic shock, which might involve this organism [138]. Decreased susceptibility to third-generation cephalosporins and resistance to other classes of antimicrobial drugs, including quinolones, may limit treatment options for invasive pneumococcal disease [177].

Microorganism lysis – caused by antibiotics– is desirable and is associated with a significant improvement of patient prognosis [178]. However, this phenomenon may be associated with significant adverse effects; indeed, 4-6 hours after the administration of large doses of antibiotics, systemic vasodilation and hypotension may occur. This effect may be the result of the release of large amounts of toxin as a result of the antibiotic-caused lysis of large numbers of microorganisms [179]. This phenomenon may be observed in gram-positive and gram-negative infection; the resulting systemic inflammatory response can be modified (and the shock decreased) in animals pretreated with steroids or non-steroidal anti-inflammatory drugs [180].

Regarding the localization of the infectious source, the lung is the most common site of infection, followed by the abdomen and urinary tract [3]. Other investigators [181] reported that the likely sources of infection leading to bacteremia and sepsis in the critically ill (trauma) patient are vascular sources (64 %), intraabdominal infection (48 %), pneumonia (38 %), wound infections (30 %), and the urinary tract (7 %). The source of infection seems to be an important determinant of clinical outcome. The greatest risk of developing severe sepsis occurs in the setting of bacteremia associated with nosocomial pneumonia [119]. Patients with intraabdominal infections and polymicrobial bacteraemia or postoperative wound infections and bacteremia are at significant risk for developing severe sepsis. Bacteremia associated with intravascular catheters or indwelling urinary catheters carries a lower risk of causing septic shock [115]. General guidelines for empiric antibiotic treatment based on source of sepsis and potential pathogens are presented in ***Table 10*** [37, 119, 182].

Source Control in the Septic Patient

When evaluating a septic patient, the first step should be the recognition of the septic source; unfortunately, this is not always easy. Clinical evaluation remains important in the diagnostic approach of the septic patient. Unfortunatelyy, it is not always helpful, especially in the critically ill, septic patient. Cultures of the blood, sputum, and urine should be obtained and a chest radiograph should be performed. Bronchoscopy may be required in patients in whom mucus plugging occurs or in patients where better sputum cultures are needed to be obtained [37, 135]. The clinician should use all the available diagnostic modalities, including the modern sophisticated imaging methods (i.e. ultrasonography and computed tomography and/or MRI) to localize the source of sepsis. Most infections in the chest involve pneumonia, but empyema or complex pneumonia, endocarditis, pericarditis, and mediastinitis may be also the cause of sepsis. The abdominal cavity is usually very difficult to evaluate, especially in critically ill patients. Potential intraabdominal causes of sepsis include cholecystitis or cholangitis, ischemic bowel, intraabdominal interloop abscesses, tubo-ovarian abscesses. Perirectal abscesses are another potential source of sepsis. Infections in the extremities, such as abscesses or septic phlebitis, and severe necrotizing soft tissue infections (such as necrotizing fasciitis and Fournier's disease) may trigger the inflammatory cascade leading to the clinical syndrome of septic shock. Central venous catheter-related infection is another consideration for the septic patient.

«Source control» is the term that describes the intervention(s) used to control the source of an infection; this intervention may be a surgical procedure (such as debridement of necrotic infected tissue back to healthy tissue, diversion or repair or excision of an ongoing focus of contamination from a perforated hollow viscus), but may also include other "simpler" measures such as removal of an infected intravascular catheter, tube thoracostomy to drain an empyema of the pleural cavity, or other minimally invasive procedures to achieve drainage of

Table 10. Empiric antibiotic selection

Common infections, causative organisms, and recommended antibiotics

Suspected source of sepsis	Causative organism	Recommended empiric therapy
Lung – CA (*)	**Streptococcus pneumonia** *Haemophilus influenzae* *Legionella* species **Chlamydia pneumoniae** *Pneumocystis carinii*	Macrolide + third-generation cephalospirin
Lung – HA (**)	Aerobic gram-negative bacilli	Cefipime or imipenem-cilastatin + aminoglycoside
Intraabdominal sepsis – CA (*)	**Escherichia coli** *Bacteroides fragilis*	Imipenem-cilastatin or Piperacillin-tazobactam ± aminoglycoside
Intraabdominal sepsis – HA (**)	Aerobic gram-negative rods Anaerobes *Candida* species	Imipenem-cilastatin ± aminoglycoside or Piperacillin-tazobactam ± amphotericin B
Skin, soft tissues, wound – CA (*)	Group A streptococcus **Staphylococcus aureus** *Clostridium* species Polymicrobial Enteric gram-negative rods *Pseudomonas aeruginosa* Anaerobes Staphylococci	Vancomycin ± Imipenem-cilastatin or Piperacillin-tazobactam
Skin, soft tissues, wound – HA (**)	**Staphylococcus aureus** Aerobic gram-negative rods	Vancomycin + Cefipime
Urinary tract – CA (*)	**Escherichia coli** *Klebsiella* species *Enterobacter* species *Proteus* species	Ciprofloxacin ± aminoglycoside
Urinary tract – HA (**)	Aerobic gram-negative rods Enterococci	Vancomycin + Cefipime
CNS – CA (*)	**Streptococcus pneumoniae** *Neisseria meningiditis* *Listeria monocytogenes* *Escherichia coli* *Haemophilus influenzae*	Vancomycin + third generation cephalosporin or meropenem

Table 10. Continued

Suspected source of sepsis	Causative organism	Recommended empiric therapy
CNS – HA (**)	**Pseudomonas aeruginosa**	Cefipime or
	Escherichia coli	Meropenem + Vancomycin
	Klebsiella species	
	Staphylococci species	
Catheter-related sepsis	**Staphylococcus aureus**	Vancomycin
	Staphylococcus epidermidis	Vancomycin
	Klebsiella species	Third generation cephalosporin or ciprofloxacin
	Enterobacter species	Imipenem or Piperacillin-tazobactam
	Serratia species	Gentamycin or third generation cephalosporin or imipenem

(*) CA = major community acquired infections
(**) HA = major nosocomial infections (hospital acquired)

infected fluid collections (for example ultrasonographically-guided percutaneous drainage of an empyema of the gallbladder, CT-guided drainage of an intraabdominal abscess, endoscopic sphincterotomy for suppurative cholangitis, etc) (see below). For these reasons, "source control" is more appropriate as a term compared to other previous terms, such as "surgical therapy", "surgery", "surgical procedure", etc [183].

The newer therapeutic approach and the shift from open surgery to minimally invasive procedures is largely due to the impressive and significant recent advances in interventional radiology; these advances have enabled us to use minimally invasive procedures to achieve source control in cases where surgery was in the past unavoidable and have simplified the management of septic patient; these radiologically guided approaches are associated with minimal morbidity and mortality and – if effective drainage can be achieved – should be preferred over open surgery, given the critical condition of patients with septic shock. The two methods (open surgery and minimally invasive therapeutic approaches) should be viewed as complementary. Indeed, open surgery will be required for a significant percentage of patients, such as those with infections involving necrotic tissue (i.e., infected necrotizing pancreatitis, necrotic soft tissue infections) and for the drainage of complex abscesses (i.e., abscesses with thick purulent material, or with septae within the abscess cavity).

Source control is of key importance in the management of the septic patient, since the presence of a remaining infectious nidus as a continuing source of infection guarantees the progression of the inflammatory cascade and the development of Multiple Organ Dysfunction / Multiple Organ Failure Syndrome (MODS / MOFS) with a resultant high mortality risk [171]. Inadequate source control is associated with a poor clinical outcome [184]. The potential indication and the role of source control should be evaluated for all patients with severe sepsis. In many circumstances – as, for example, the patient with diffuse peritonitis from a perforated ulcer or clostridial myonecrosis following a traumatic injury - the need for source control of the septic source is clear. Obviously, surgical elimination of the septic focus is not always possible; a typical example are the septic patients with pneumonia, where tracheal sunctioning and physiotherapy to enhance elimination of contaminated secretions are source control measures that may be of benefit. As noted above, early administration of the appropriate antimicrobial agents is particularly important where the septic focus cannot be removed.

Clinical judgment is required to determine the optimal timing of intervention. The benefits of intervention in providing definitive control of a focus of infection should be balanced against the risks of an interventional procedure. Usually, such treatment should proceed as soon as the diagnosis has been made, delaying only to correct immediately remediable electrolytic disturbances, severe anemia, and cardiorespiratory instability. Many of these patients are necessarily at high operative risk because of their critical general condition. However, if the infective process is a major cause of their unstable condition, and surgical therapy is required to correct it, delaying intervention in the hope that medical treatment will lead to the surgery being done under more favorable conditions is usually an error and results in worsening of the general condition of the patient [185].

Necrotizing Fasciitis

Streptococcus spp and Clostridium spp are usually the main responsible microorganisms [186]. Necrotizing fasciitis typically occurs in a normal host approximately 50 years of age; however, these infections can occur in young patients with a very minor traumatic injury that is just barely remembered. The disease process evolves through a spectrum of stages; it usually starts as cellulites and then severe infection occurs, by burrowing down into the soft tissues and by spreading into the fascial planes. Every effort should be made to recognize severe infection and to distinguish an infection that is limited to the subcutaneous tissue and may respond to antibiotic therapy alone (cellulitis) from an infection causing necrosis of deep fat, muscle fascia, and muscle (necrotizing fasciitis) that needs aggressive intervention (debridement). At the early phase of the disease process, this distinction may be very difficult. Necrotizing soft tissue infections may be associated with normal skin, and local signs may be mild, despite the presence of extensive deeper tissue necrosis [183]. Extensive soft tissue edema, crepitus, and cyanosis or bronzing of the skin is late presentations. A high index of suspicion is required for early recognition of the disease. There are some keys that can be used in an effort to early diagnose severe deep necrotizing infection: pain and fever out of proportion to the physical findings (since this is a toxin-mediated disease) and a very high blood cell count [187]. The diagnosis can be confirmed by imaging studies such as CT or MRI, which are very useful in showing subcutaneous tissue gas and/or thickening of the fascia, or retroperitoneal extension, or even non-enhancement of tissues following administration of intravenous contrast [183, 188]. When the diagnosis is confirmed, the patient should be taken immediately to the operating room. Surgical therapy consists in a wide resection of all nonviable tissues back to healthy tissue. Especially for muscle necrosis, fascial compartments must be opened to relieve the increased pressure within the muscle compartment (compartment syndrome) and to allow an adequate blood supply to the muscle. In many of these patients with severe necrotizing soft tissue infections reoperations may be necessary to obtain adequate debridement of newly necrosed tissue formed as a result of an ongoing severe infection [37, 135]. When there is any doubt, it is best to make an incision and look for the presence of tissue necrosis. Since the tissue is necrotic, it does not bleed. The first 4 – 6 hours of the natural course of necrotizing fasciitis are critical for the prognosis of the patient. Ideally, surgical debridement should be performed within 3 h or – at least – 12 h of admission [189, 190]. Delaying the intervention may result in the death of the patient from extensive disease [191]. It should be emphasized that the morbidity of surgical exploration is extremely low. If surgical exploration is negative, the patient has simply an incision without debridement; however, if the finding is positive, then early exploratory surgery is an important step to control the development of the whole disease. At surgery, all infected, devitalized, or non-bleeding soft tissue should be removed. Inadequate resection of necrotic tissue, as well as delaying surgery, results in increased mortality [192].

Antibiotics should be given in patients with severe soft tissue infections (serious cellulitis or deep necrotizing infection) in high doses and early. In selecting the antibiotic regimen, it should be remembered that the majority of patients with necrotizing fasciitis have polymicrobial infections and typically these mixed infections consist of gram-positive cocci (usually spaphylococci), aerobic gram-negative bacilli, and anaerobes. High dose penicillin, a very broad-spectrum agent such as meropenem, and clindamycin are indicated in these cases.

If Clostridium spp is the responsible microorganism, clindamycin stops the production of A toxin. If the patient is diabetic, injection drug user, or if the infection has an abdominal presentation, probably complexe microbiology is present and the antibiotic regimen should be directed toward these potential pathogens [193, 194]. Subsequent antibiotic therapy should be based on the findings of culture.

In a recently described syndrome, severe soft tissue infection - the so-called idiopathic necrotizing fasciitis - may be caused by group A streptococci without an obvious portal of entry and no break in the skin. It has been hypothesized that infection is spread to soft tissue by hematogenous spread (metastatic infection) from unknown sources, perhaps the oropharynx [195, 196].

Fournier's Disease

Is a necrotizing infection of the perineum, caused by both aerobes and anaerobes microorganisms (polymicrobial synergistic infection). A black spot on the scrotum is a pathognomonic sign in the early course of Fournier's disease. Again, as in necrotizing fasciitis, disproportionate pain and fever and an elevated blood cell count are typically observed in Fournier's disease [197]. Management should be the same as in severe soft tissue infections (wide resection of nonviable tissues and appropriate antibiotic therapy). If substantial dissection is necessary, a proximal diverting colostomy may improve wound healing [198].

Perirectal Abscesses

Perirectal abscesses may be an ominous source of infection in the septic patient and an often-misunderstood form of infection, especially in patients with diabetes or in patients with an altered immune function (for example patients receiving corticosteroids or chemotherapy) [183, 197]. The typical fluctuance may not be observed. Pain on defecation and induration in the area are useful diagnostic clues. Needle aspiration usually yields purulent material, thereby establishing the diagnosis. The definitive management of perirectal abscesses is prompt surgical intervention. Antibiotics should be used only as an adjunct. Wide surgical drainage should be performed in the operating room, under adequate anesthesia. Treatment failures in patients with perirectal abscesses are those in whom the abscess is not recognized, is inadequately drained (for example in complex abscesses with intracavitary septae), or in whom treatment consists of antimicrobial agents alone [197].

Toxic Shock Syndrome

Toxic shock syndrome (or menstrual toxic shock) is a rare infection characterized by fever, erythematous rash, desquamation of the palms and soles of the feet late in the course of the disease, hypotention, and eventually multiple organ failure. Although originally this syndrome was described in women having a tampon in the vagina for a long time, there are now surgical wound infections linked to this type of severe infection [197, 199]. The main causative microorgarnism is S. aureus and patients who do not have antibodies against toxic shock syndrome toxin-1 are susceptible for the development of this syndrome. Toxic shock syndrome may also be caused by streptococci [200]. Commonly, the toxic shock is not an invasive infection, since the responsible microorganism proliferates in the foreign body (tampon). Indeed, only 3 % of patients with toxic shock have blood cultures positive for staphylococci. In contrast, 80 % of patients will have a positive blood culture with the invasive group A streptococci [201].

It should be emphasized that the wound that is the cause of toxic shock can look extremely innocent. It can be a simple hematoma that later gets infected through the blood stream and does on to produce the potentially lethal toxin [197, 201]. Treatment is symptomatic; the tampon should be removed, the wound should be drained, and antibiotics should be given to suppress the offending microorganism [201].

Intraabdominal Abscesses

Diagnosis of an intraabdominal pathology, such as intraabdominal abscess, as a cause of septic shock is not easy in the severely ill patient. Clinical examination may be unreliable, especially if the patient is under mechanical ventilation. In order to accurately diagnose an intraabdominal abscess the clinician should rely on modern imaging methods (ultrasonography and CT). Despite some disadvantages (such as being operator dependent, inability to image a pathology in the presence of significant amounts of gas within the intestinal lumen or in the presence of external dressings or drains etc), ultrasonography remains an extremely useful diagnostic toll for the initial evaluation of the septic patient [202, 203]. It can be performed at the bedside in the ICU therefore obviating the transport of the critically ill patient to the CT department. Moreover, a well-trained radiologist can aspirate a fluid collection or insert a catheter for percutaneous therapeutic drainage of an abscess under ultrasonographic guidance. However, due to the above - mentioned limitations of ultrasonography. abdominal computed tomography (CT) remains the "gold standard" in the diagnostic approach of a patient with a possible intraabdominal source of infection (such as intra-abdominal abscess or infected necrotic pancreatic or peripancreatic tissue).

CT has a high sensitivity and specificity for the diagnosis of foci of infection and can delineate with impressive anatomic accuracy its location [204, 205]. Additionally, CT can be used to guide diagnostic (i.e., fine needle aspiration [FNA] to obtain sample for microbiological analysis in necrotizing acute pancreatitis) or therapeutic procedures (i.e., drainage of infected fluid collection). When an intravenous contrast agent is given, CT can differentiate viable and non-viable tissue (contrast-enhanced or "dynamic" computed tomography). To differentiate intraluminal intestinal fluids from other pathologic fluid collections oral gastrographin should be given 1 – 2 hours prior the examination. CT is extremely useful for the imaging of the retroperitoneum, an anatomic area where the limitations of ultrasonography are well known.

Other less commonly used today radiological studies may be used in selected cases. A typical example is the administration of a water-soluble contrast agent (i.e., gastrographin) to delineate the site of perforation of a hollow viscus (such as esophagus, duodenum, sigmoid etc) and to image the collection of fluid within a cavity. In the past, sinography (injection of gastrographin through a drain) was used to demonstrate the presence of a residual abscess cavity and any possible connection of the sinus with the gastrointestinal tract. Nowadays, many of this information can be obtained from the abdominal CT; for example, in the case of a perforation of a hollow viscus CT will show the presence of air within the abdomen and the presence of fluid in the area adjacent to the site of perforation [205].

Appropriate early drainage is the best treatment. The early use of parenteral antibiotics aimed at colonic aerobes and anaerobes, or antibiotics effective against identified (cultured) pathogen(s) is usually necessary [197]. The drainage can be performed either percutaneously or surgically. Percutaneous drainage, if it can be performed effectively, is generally preferable to surgical intervention and should be considered as the treatment of choice in patients with localized intraabdominal abscess without signs of generalized peritonitis [183, 197]. In favorable cases, such as unilocular, well-defined fluid collections, for which a safe drainage route could be easily established, success rate is impressive (up to 92 %) [206]. However, indications and access routes for percutaneous drainage have been recently expanded and include intraabdominal abscesses complicating diseases such as diverticulitis, pancreatitis, appendicitis, or abscesses observed during the postoperative period. For example, for intraabdominal abscesses complicating colorectal procedures, the primary success was 65% after the first and 85% after a second drainage [207]. Multiple, ill-defined abscesses, abscesses communicating with the gastrointestinal tract, or abscesses whose drainage would require a route through normal organs (i.e. liver) can be treated percutaneously with as success rate of 74 % [208].

Percutaneous drainage has many advantages compared to surgical drainage, such as lower invasiveness and cost, almost equal efficiency, elimination of the contamination of surrounding tissues, obviation of the need for postoperative wound management, and avoidance of the later risks of incisional hernia, a possible complication especially if the wound becomes infected postoperatively [209]. Even if percutaneous catheter drainage cannot achieve complete drainage of the abscess, it can be used as a temporising measure to optimise the physiologic and hemodynamic condition of an acutely/severely ill patient prior to a second attempt for percutaneous drainage or a definitive surgical operation [183].

It is important to emphasize that percutaneous drainage and surgical drainage techniques should not be considered competitive but rather complementary. If an abscess is accessible by percutaneous techniques, it is reasonable to consider a non-operative approach to the problem, particularly for the critically ill, septic patient. It is also clear that patients should respond promptly to whatever technique is employed to drain their intra-abdominal abscess. An improvement should be seen clinically within 24 to 48 hours following drainage. Should improvement not be forthcoming, the patient must be aggressively re-evaluated with repeat CT and decisions made by the responsible surgeon in consultation with the radiologist as to the next appropriate course of action. Patients are rarely too sick for an appropriate operation. Although most abscesses can be successfully treated by percutaneous drainage, open surgery should be performed when there are no well-defined collections, when dead tissues require debridement, or when residual collections cannot be treated percutaneously [183]. Such examples include pancreatic abscesses with pancreatic necrosis that generally require surgical debridement, usually accompanied by repeated explorations (see below). Another indication of open surgery is when there is a source of ongoing peritoneal contamination (such as a perforated hollow viscus). Even splenic abscesses, once considered as a contraindication for percutaneous drainage, can today safely be drained percutaneously, under image-guidance; this method is currently considered as a safe and effective alternative to open surgery, allowing preservation of the spleen [210].

Severe (Necrotic) Acute Pancreatitis

In most cases (~ 80 %), acute pancreatitis is mild and self-limiting, subsiding within 3 – 5 days. Mild acute pancreatitis should be managed conservatively. Severe, necrotizing pancreatitis develops in about 20 % of cases; in these cases, parts of the pancreatic parenchyma and / or peripancreatic tissues become necrotic. The natural course of necrotic pancreatitis is characterized by two phases. The first phase evolves during the first two weeks after the onset of symptoms the disease and is characterized by the systemic inflammatory response syndrome (SIRS). It is important to emphasize that SIRS in the early phase of severe pancreatitis may be found in the absence of significant pancreatic necrosis and is frequently found in the absence of pancreatic infection [211]. The second phase is characterized by the development of infection of pancreatic necrosis; that usually develops after the first two weeks following the onset of symptoms. It has been estimated that infection of the necrotic pancreatic tissues develops in as many as 40 – 70 % of patients with necrotizing pancreatitis [212]. The risk of infection increases with the extent of intra- and extra-pancreatic necrosis [213]. Even with the use of prophylactic antibiotic therapy, infection of pancreatic necrosis is still a major risk factor in severe pancreatitis, whilst sepsis-related multiple organ failure is the main life-threatening complication with a mortality rate of 20 – 50 % [214]. It has been showed that the use of prophylactic broad-spectrum antibiotics reduces infection rates in CT-proven necrotizing pancreatitis, but may not improve survival.

Contrast-enhanced ("dynamic') CT scan is the method of choice for the diagnosis of pancreatic necrosis. Once pancreatic necrosis has developed, the differentiation between sterile and infected necrosis is essential for the management of patients. Image (US or CT)-guided fine-needle aspiration (FNA) for bacteriology of pancreatic or peripancreatic necrosis has been established as an accurate, safe and reliable technique for the identification of infected necrosis [215] and is indicated in patients who develop significant pancreatic necrosis and clinical signs of sepsis.

Proven infected pancreatic necrosis as well as septic complications directly resulting from pancreatic infection are indications for intervention including surgery and radiological drainage [216, 217]. The conservative management of infected pancreatic necrosis associated with multiple organ failure has a mortality rate of up to 100 % [218]. In contrast, the surgical treatment of patients with infected pancreatic necrosis is associated with a much better prognosis and some specialized centers have reported mortality rates as low as 10 – 30 % [219 - 221]. Debridement of infected devitalized pancreatic and/or peripancreatic tissue is a critical element in source control, eliminating a locus of unopposed microbial growth. Necrotic tissues offer an excellent culture medium for microorganisms and – given the lack of blood supply - bacterial proliferation is possible in an environment that is protected from host inflammatory cells.

While infected pancreatic necrosis is a clear indication for surgery, the benefits of excising uninfected necrotic pancreatic tissue are less clear, and must be weighted against the risks of attempted excision. Most patients with sterile necrosis respond to conservative non-surgical medical management [219]. Nevertheless, some patients do not improve despite maximal therapy in the ICU and the role of surgery remains debatable in those patients who develop organ failure associated with sterile pancreatic necrosis [222, 223]. Fulminant acute pancreatitis is characterized by rapidly progressive multiple organ failure in the first few days following the onset of acute pancreatitis with a high probability of death despite ICU therapy; in fulminant acute pancreatitis, prognosis remains dismal with both surgical and conservative therapies [224, 225].

Regarding the optimal timing of surgery, it should be emphasized that in the early stages of tissue necrosis (1st and 2nd week), viable tissue is not clearly demarcated from non-viable tissue, and an intermediate zone of hyperemic inflammatory tissue is present; bleeding during attempted excision at this early stage may be considerable and this is an important reason that delayed debridement of infected pancreatic necrosis is associated with a better clinical outcome [226]. With time, the demarcation of viable from non-viable tissue becomes cleared, and intervention is facilitated; for this reason surgery in severe acute pancreatitis should be deferred whilst the patient continues to respond positively to conservative management. The 3rd and 4th week after the onset of the disease is generally agreed to provide the optimal operative conditions for necrosectomy, with the effect of limiting the extent of surgery that is needed to facilitate debridement. This approach decreases the risk of bleeding and minimizes the surgery-related endocrine loss of vital pancreatic tissue that predisposes to surgery-induced endocrine and exocrine pancreatic insufficiency. At surgery, all areas of necrotic and infected tissue should be removed. The aim is to reduce the process of spreading necrosis and/or infection and the release of proinflammatory mediators. An organ-preserving approach is indicated; following debridement or necrosectomy a postoperative management aiming to maximize postoperative evacuation of retroperitoneal debris and exudates is indicated. The role of percutaneous techniques remains relatively limited to some subgroups of patients such as those with localized and/or well-organized pancreatic necrosis; however, a certain number of these patients will require subsequent laparotomy to control sepsis [227, 228].

Specific operative approaches (such as continuous postoperative peritoneal lavage, or open abdomen) have been proposed for the management of patients with infected pancreatic necrosis. Although favorable results with these aggressive surgical techniques have been reported [219 - 221, 229], there is no conclusive evidence about the superiority of these methods over the conventional surgical technique. Current data support the concept that relaparotomy "on demand" as indicated by worsening of the clinical status, absence of improvement, or evolving organ dysfunction is as efficacious as these more aggressive approach [183]. Planned relaparotomy is indicated when intestinal viability is a concern ("second look"), for patients with necrotizing pancreatitis when demarcation of necrotic tissue demarcation is not distinct, or when bleeding precludes complete debridement.

Specifically regarding gallstone-associated acute pancreatitis, cholecystectomy should be performed to avoid recurrence of the disease; in mild acute pancreatitis cholecystectomy should be performed as soon as the patient has recovered and ideally during the same hospital admission. In contrast, in severe gallstone-associated acute pancreatitis, cholecystectomy should be delayed until there is sufficient resolution of the inflammatory response and clinical recovery [217]. Endoscopic sphincterotomy is an alternative to cholecystectomy in those who are not fit to undergo surgery in order to lower the risk of recurrence of biliary pancreatitis. There is, however, a theoretical risk of introducing infection into sterile pancreatic necrosis [216, 217].

Foreign Body-Related Infections

The insertion of implants and medical devices is a commonly performed and often a life-saving procedure. It has been estimated that the rate of total hip replacement in a worldwide basis is approximately one million a year, and knee replacements more than 250.000. More than 30 % of hospitalized patients have one or more vascular catheters in place and more than 10 % of hospitalized patients have an indwelling urinary catheter [230]. The presence of a foreign body (for example a retained surgical sponge) or an invasive medical device (such an intravascular catheter, a prosthetic cardiac valve, an orthopedic implant, etc) is one of the most important risk factor for the development of sepsis. The foreign body predisposes to infection by damaging or invading epithelial or mucosal barriers, and by protecting micro-organisms from the host defenses, thus serving as reservoirs resulting in resistant chronic infection or tissue necrosis. Tissue damage caused by surgery and foreign body implantation further increases the susceptibility to infections, activates host defenses and stimulates the generation of inflammatory mediators; these are enhanced by bacterial activity and toxins. Some microorganisms, such as coagulase-negative Staphylococci, form biofilms on prosthetic materials that permit the establishment of microbial colonies, and protect the bacteria from host immune cells [231]. Interestingly, in the presence of a foreign body, the number of microorganisms required to establish a focus of infection is significantly reduced [232]. Currently, implant devices account for approximately half (~50 %) of all nosocomial infections.

Implant infections are extremely resistant to antibiotics and host defenses and frequently persist until the implant is removed, which is the standard therapy and an important step in the process of source control. Again, however, the clinician must balance risks and benefits. When the infected foreign body is a retained surgical sponge or a colonized Foley catheter, the decision to remove the foreign body is obvious. Removal of an infected mesh following herniorrhaphy is not an easy procedure and may be associated with significant complications, especially in large postoperative hernias. Removal of a prosthetic heart valve, a vascular graft, or even a peritoneal dialysis catheter in a patient with dialysis-dependent renal failure entails an ever greater degree of risk; in these cases, an intensive trial of non-interventional management in needed [183].

Central line related infection is the most common cause of S. aureus bacteremia in hospitalized patients. Gram-negative bacteria, such as enterobacter, Pseudomonas, Acinetobacter, and Candida species are frequently isolated in catheter-related infection. Patients with severe sepsis without an obvious source of infection should have central venous catheter removed; the tip of the catheter should be send for culture. The diagnosis of a catheter-related bacteremia is based on the isolation of the same microorganism from the tip of the catheter (intravascular portion) and the blood. The number of microorganisms cultured at the tip of the catheter should be large enough to consider the catheter as the main source of bacteremia (see below). Moreover, clinical and microbiological information should rule out another site of infection. A semiquantitative technique to differentiate contamination of a catheter from true infection was described [233, 234]. In this method, the distal part of the catheter (~ 5 cm) is cultured and blood cultures are taken from other sites, at a distance from the point of entry of the catheter. A catheter-related infection is diagnosed when more than 15 CFU are cultured from the tip of the catheter but blood cultures are negative. Catheter-related bacteremia is diagnosed when more than 15 CFU are cultured from the tip of the catheter and the same microorganism is diagnosed in the cultures of the peripheral blood. Finally, bacteremia of another etiologies should be considered if less than 15 CFU are cultured from the tip of the catheter and the same microorganism is cultured in the peripheral blood. The semiquantitative method has a sensitivity of 36 % and a specificity of 100 %. An infected central venous catheter can be safely changed using a guidewire, provided there is no significant local tissue infection at the exit site. This technique is associated with fewer mechanical complications compared to replacement at a new site; its disadvantage is a higher probability that the new catheter will become infected at the exit-site [235]. Empiric antibiotic therapy with vancomycin and an extended spectrum cephalosporin or aminoglycoside should be initiated. Subsequent antibiotic therapy should be based on the results of cultures. If fever and bacteremia persist, evaluation for endocarditis, septic thrombophlebitis, or a metastatic focus of infection (originated from the infected central venous line) such as septic arthritis, should be undertaken [236].

Tunneled silastic catheters, such as the Hickman or Broviac catheter, are associated with a lower rate of infection. An extensive tunnel infection, evidenced by the presence of erythema, induration or purulence along the subcutaneous tract, is an indication for catheter removal, while exit-site infections (clinical evidence of infection within 2 cm of the exit site) should be managed conservatively (local wound care plus appropriate antibiotic therapy) [237]. Peripheral septic thrombophlebitis is quite uncommon. In this case, the catheter should be removed and the infected vein excised, leaving the wound open to heal by the formation of granulation tissue [238].

In an attempt to reduce the incidence of catheter-related infections, a number of approaches have been proposed. Routine catheter replacement not only failed to reduce the risk of catheter-related bacteremia, but also was associated with a higher incidence of catheter-related infection [239]. At most hospitals, central venous catheters are changed when evidence of infection is present (signs of inflammation, purulent discharge at the insertion site) or when there are indications that the lumen of the catheter is partially or totally obstructed [235, 239, 240]. The ability of bacteria such as Staphylococcus epidermidis, which are otherwise virtually avirulent, to escape from host defences and antibiotic therapy, has led to the development of infection-resistant materials acting as antimicrobial drug-delivery systems. By these methods, there is a sustained delivery of antimicrobial drugs into the local microenvironment of implants, which avoids systemic side effects and exceeds usual systemic concentrations by several orders of magnitude. Bioengineering of hybrid implant materials in order to achieve optimal performance and to prevent inflammatory reactions and interface cellular disorganization is a field undergoing rapid development. Hybrid materials that slowly deliver antimicrobial drugs may reduce implant infections in the future [230].

Other Causes of Acute Abdomen

Early diagnosis and treatment of intra-abdominal pathology in critically ill intensive care unit (ICU) patients remains a clinical challenge [185, 241]. The mortality rate is closely related to the delay in surgical evaluation and intervention. This emphasizes again the crucial role of timely surgical intervention in treating acute abdomen [241, 242]. Absence of typical clinical findings because of altered mental state, medications, immunosuppression, or underlying disease, has long been recognized as a reason for a delay in surgical evaluation and intervention [243]. High clinical suspicion, repeated abdominal examinations, radiologic investigation, and most importantly, early surgical involvement, are recommended to reduce the significant mortality rates associated with surgical delay [242]. In a recent study from the Mayo Clinic [241], about 95 % of patients with acute abdomen at a medical ICU have some abdominal tenderness on physical examination; however, only 38 % demonstrated peritoneal signs. In this study, absence of peritoneal signs was associated – as expected - with surgical delay. The unreliability of physical examination in these critically ill patients can explain why the surgeon should be based on other diagnostic modalities. Abdominal computed tomography (CT) is the procedure of choice for the diagnostic evaluation of the septic patient with suspected intraabdominal pathology. Abdominal CT has a higher sensitivity for the detection of free air compared with plain radiographs [241, 244]. In the absence of free air, however, CT findings (bowel wall thickening, ileus, ascites) are of low sensitivity and specificity [245]. Especially difficult is the diagnostic evaluation of the critically ill patient with underlying ischemic bowel. Abdominal ultrasound is particularly useful in the diagnosis of gallbladder disease (where it is more sensitive than the CT scanning). However, the specificity and sensitivity of ultrasound is very low in other clinical situations, thereby limiting its utility in critically ill patients [246].

Bedside abdominal paracentesis, diagnostic peritoneal lavage (DPL), and diagnostic laparoscopy have been proposed as useful diagnostic tools in the evaluation of septic patient with potential acute abdomen. Abdominal paracentesis may be performed in the presence of ascitis; it can also be performed when there is a suspicion for a perforation of a hollow viscus when radiologic studies are non-diagnostic. DPL is safe but has relatively low sensitivity [247]. DPL can be performed under ultrasound or CT guidance if there is a localized fluid collection. Bedside laparoscopy may be of help in selected patients, but its safety and sensitivity need to be defined [241]. The procedure may be difficult outside the operating room in most hospital settings. In predicting the need for laparotomy, laparoscopy was more accurate than DPL [247].

It is well known that some milder cases of acute abdomen in the septic patient may resolve without surgical intervention; such typical cases are mild episodes of acute cholecystitis, acute appendicitis, diverticulitis, etc. In these cases probably the surgical problem is not the cause of the septic shock and therefore other etiologies should be excluded. The clinician should focus on abdominal "catastrophes", conditions invariably fatal without prompt surgical intervention. In these cases, prompt intervention – as indicated – is necessary for an effective source control. Ideally, this is accomplished by surgical removal of the involved structure; for example, appendectomy for acute perforated appendicitis or cholecystectomy for gangrenous acute cholecystitis. Drainage alone can serve to create a controlled fistula, and it is frequently a less morbid interim (temporary) solution, allowing a stabilization of the critical general condition of the septic patient. Effective minimally invasive procedures are reasonable alternatives for critically ill patients with selected diseases. Percutaneous, image-guided cholecystostomy is a minimally invasive procedure, easy to perform, with low complication and high success rates that can be used as the procedure of choice in patients with acute cholecystitis unfit for emergency surgery. Patients often improve clinically, so that cholecystectomy can be done electively. Interestingly, percutaneous cholecystostomy may be definitive treatment, especially in acalculous cholecystitis [248, 249]. Endoscopic sphincterotomy (ES) is the treatment of choice for (severe) acute cholangitis, especially for critically ill, septic patients [250]. Open common bile duct exploration is rarely indicated today, and should be considered only in selected cases, such as for management of severe complications after ES as perforations of the duodenum, large common bile duct stones and patients with Mirizzi's syndrome or intrahepatic stones with stenosis of the bile duct [250]. When acute abdomen is due to a perforation of a hollow viscus, abdominal contamination can be reduced by proximal diversion or defunctioning of the perforated viscus. For example, in mediastinitis secondary to an intrathoracic rupture of the esophagus, mediastinal drainage and the creation of a cervical esophagostomy are indicated. Drainage of the abscess and a colostomy created proximal to a colonic perforation (secondary to cancer or diverticulitis) are indicated, therefore reducing the volume of gastrointestinal effluent passing across the injured colon and thus minimizing the leakage of bacteria into tissues surrounding the perforation. However, this principle is not applicable in all the cases of perforations of the gastrointestinal tract; for example, currently standard therapy for a perforated peptic ulcer consists simply of an omental patch with or without an acid-reducing procedure. It should be emphasized that simple drainage and diversion – although technically simpler - leaves the source of contamination in place; currently, there is a clear trend to resect – when possible - the diseased perforated viscus during the first procedure. A typical example of this strategy is colonic perforation secondary to a sigmoid colon cancer or diverticulitis, where a Hartman procedure is a reasonable and preferable option (excision of the diseased part of the colon, with closure of the peripheral stump and creation of an end-colostomy). Iatrogenic perforations of a hollow viscus are associated with a better prognosis [251, 252]. Due to the preparation of the colon prior to the diagnostic procedure (i.e., colonoscopy), the surgeon has more choices in these cases, including simple suture of the perforation – if applicable – which is typically contraindicated in an unprepared colon. Ischemic bowel is a diagnostic challenge for the clinician. Resection of non-viable bowel is indicated and frequently these patients are re-operated to make sure that the remaining bowel is viable. However, the prognosis of patients with ischemic bowel remains dismal [241, 243].

In selecting the optimal surgical procedure, the surgeon should take into consideration the general condition of the patient. The additional operative time for a more complicated procedure (i.e., excision vs. simple diversion) and the resulting physiological stress to a critically ill patient may increase perioperative morbidity and mortality. However, for the majority of patients, resection is associated with lower morbidity, a shorter hospital stay and period of disability and a higher rate of colostomy reversal. Clinical judgment is required from the part of the astute clinician to select the optimal procedure for the individual patient.

Exploratory Laparotomy in the Critically Ill Septic Patient

Acute abdominal complications are perceived as relatively common events in the ICU and have been regarded as a "silent offender" because of the absence of typical clinical signs and symptoms [253]. As is well known, uncontrolled / occult infection is associated with the septic shock and the development of the multiple organ failure syndrome. This stimulated in the past the interest for the concept of "blind" exploratory laparotomy undertaken in the absence of radiological evidence of infection to search for an undrained abscess [185, 254 - 256]. However, improved radiological techniques (mainly computed tomography) have tempered the initial enthusiasm for this approach. There is no evidence that empirical or "blind" exploratory laparotomy in the critically ill patient improves outcome. Indeed, intraabdominal infections mandating source control are almost always evident using modern diagnostic imaging techniques. Nowadays, there is little if any role for empirical laparotomy to rule out undiagnosed infection in a critically ill patient in whom evaluation using the modern imaging methods (ultrasonography and particularly CT) has failed to demonstrate a surgically correctable problem. Significant occult pathology is relatively uncommon, and when encountered there is no evidence that a more aggressive approach alters outcome [185, 256, 257].

Following any attempt for eliminating the source of infection, the physician should try to evaluate the results of his/her intervention (see below, monitoring of shock). The intervention is deemed as effective when the general condition of the patient is improved, the clinical signs of sepsis or systemic inflammation are resolving, the wound shows signs of normal healing with the formation of viable granulation tissue and re-epithelization (for example, following debridement in necrotizing fasciitis), improvement of the function of dysfunctioning organ systems, and radiographic and bacteriological indications of resolution of the septic focus. If there is any concern about the adequacy and the effectiveness of source control, a reoperation should be considered. A typical example is the reoperation for severe, necrotizing soft tissue infections, under general anesthesia, and repeat debridement until there is evidence of healthy granulation tissue throughout the wound [183]. Planned reoperation may also be indicated for patients with diffuse intestinal ischemia (to ensure bowel viability), in patients with acute narcotizing pancreatitis (see above), etc.

Nutritional Support of the Septic Patient

Protein and calorie requirements are high in the septic patient and underlying malnutrition is prevalent in patients with sepsis [258]. Of course, nutritional support does not alter the evolution of the underlying disease to sepsis and eventually to MODS / MOFS, but can effectively control single nutrient and generalized nutrient deficiency. With adequate nutritional support, reductions in morbidity and mortality have been observed [258, 259]. Hemodynamic stability should be achieved before the beginning of nutritional support. A brief period (up to several days) without nutrition is unlikely to have a serious adverse effect. There is a large body of evidence suggesting that early aggressive enteral feeding is superior to the parenteral route in reducing the morbidity and mortality in critically ill septic patients [258 - 261]. The axioma "When the tube digestive function, utilize-it!" [262, 263] should be applied in the nutritional support of the septic patient. Therefore, hemodynamically stable patients who have not recently undergone abdominal surgery can usually be fed enterally, even if bowel sounds are diminished or some abdominal distention is present [263]. The advantage of enteral as compared with parenteral feeding include gastric pH buffering, avoidance of the use of parenteral-nutrition catheters, preservation of gut mucosa, avoidance of the introduction of bacterial and toxins from the gastrointestinal tract into the circulation (preservation of the mucosa barrier function of the intestinal epithelium), a more physiologic pattern of enteric hormone secretion, the ability to administer a complete nutritional mixture including fiber, and lower cost [259 - 264]. Enteral nutrition also supports the integrity of the upper gastrointestinal tract and may obviate the need for other agents that are used to prevent stress-related gastrointestinal bleeding [16, 263, 264].

However, despite the numerous advantages of enteric nutritional support, parenteral nutrition will eventually be required in a significant percentage of critically ill patients with sepsis, for a variety of reasons, such as recent intraabdominal surgical operation or development of a surgical complication following abdominal surgery (i.e., leakage from the anastomosis following low anterior resection). Interestingly, after major trauma or sepsis the gut absorptive capacity may be decreased [265, 266].

An estimation of energy requirements can be made using the Harris-Benedict equation of basal energy expenditure (BEE) [267]:

BEE (men) = 660 + (13.7 x W) + (5.0 x H) – (6.8 x A) (in Kcal / day)
BEE (women) = 655.0 + (9.6 x W) + (1.8 x H) – (4.7 x A)
TEE = BEE x (activity factor) x (stress factor), where:
TEE = total energy expenditure, W = weight in kgr, H = height in cm, A = age in yrs
Activity factor = 1,2 for bedridden, 1.3 for ambulatory
Stress factor = 1,2 mild, 1,5 moderate, 1,8 – 2,5 severe hypermetabolism (applies for septic patients).

Another method uses parameters obtained from indirect calorimetry. This is a more sophisticated method; however, it is not widely available in clinical practice.

During starvation, protein requirements is estimated to be 1 gr / kgr /day. If an increase of the lean body mass is desirable, protein requirements should be estimated at 1.5 gr / kgr /day. In septic patients, protein requirements are increased depending to the level of stress and their protein demands may reach 2.5 gr / kgr / day [268]. However, protein should not be administered at levels above 3 gr/kgr body weight, because serious complications may appear. The ratio of non-protein calories to nitrogen depends on the level of stress (1 gr nitrogen / 150 – 200 non-protein calories for level 0, 1 gr nitrogen / 100 – 150 non-protein calories for level 1, 1 gr nitrogen / 100 non-protein calories for level 2, and 1 gr nitrogen / 80 non-protein calories for level 3) [269]. The provision of fat as a fuel source should reach its limit of tolerance to afford minimal alveolar ventilation for elimination of CO_2. Fat should not exceed 2 gr / kgr /day to avoid serious complications. Finally, given the deficient peripheral fat and glucose use in patients with sepsis, the optimal carbohydrate / fat ratio is approximately 1:2 [270].

The importance of specific nutritional components (e.g., nucleic acids, glutamine, and n-3 fatty acids) remains unproven [271].

Future Perspectives

Obviously, the persistently high mortality of sepsis and septic shock of about 40 to 60 % necessitates urgent new and effective therapeutic efforts in addition to the causal approaches of focus elimination, anti-infectious therapy with antibiotics, and supportive treatment of organ dysfunction. This can explain the strong interest for experimental methods for the management of septic shock.

Cytokine Inactivation

There is a variety of approaches for blocking cytokine action, including neutralizing cytokines that have already been produced and modulating the end-organ effects of cytokines [272 - 274]. This experimental therapeutic strategy aims at blunting / down regulating the host immune response to bacterial infection and has been proposed in an effort to improve the results of therapy of septic patients. An in-depth knowledge of the pathophysiology of septic shock is required to understand the biological basis of these experimental treatments. Unfortunately, this approach provided little clinical benefit to date and may sometimes actually be harmful [272 - 276]. One reason for this failure is that by the time a patient is recognized as having sepsis cytokines already have been produced and have induced their biologic responses. Therefore, blocking the actions of cytokines is successful if given before exercising their biologic actions. Another reason for the failure of this approach is that in septic shock multiple cellular activation and complex processes are involved and many humoral cascades are triggered [37, 171], and therefore the blockage of a single component may be insufficient to arrest the inflammatory process. Moreover, the disparate biological processes that comprise inflammation are intimately interrelated, and strategies directed at one manifestation may have significant and unexpected consequences for others. The lack of precise immunological monitoring during the course of sepsis may be an additional reason for the failure of cytokine inactivation in the management of septic shock; this lack deprives the possibility for a targeted intervention leading to a more successful immunomodulation in sepsis.

Antiendotoxin Therapy

Early trials of antiendotoxin therapy with the human and murine monoclonal antibodies against endotoxin demonstrated a decrease in the development of MODS [277]. However, the role of antiendotoxin therapy in the prevention of MODS failed to be confirmed in subsequent studies [278].

Complement Activation Blockade

Complement activation following shock and sepsis is well known and the C_{5a} fragment of the complement is implicated as a particularly potent mediator of the inflammatory process [279]. Antibodies directed against C_{5a} showed a protective effect against LPS-induced lung injury, prevented C_{5a}-induced neutropenia and apoptosis, decreased the frequency of bacteremia, and improved survival in non-human primates [280 - 282]. However, the clinical usefulness of this approach remains unproven.

Filtration

The theoretical basis for this therapeutic strategy is the removal of the inflammatory mediators from the circulation by filtration (hemofiltration or plasma filtration). Given the central role of these noxious substances in the pathophysiology of septic shock, their elimination may influence outcome of critically ill, septic patients [283 - 286]. The role of filtration is clear in septic patients with acute renal failure. Interestingly, daily dialysis (as compared with traditional every other day or intermittent dialysis) significantly reduced mortality (28 % for daily dialysis vs. 46 % for alternate-day dialysis, $p=0.01$) [287]. Of note, increased morbidity secondary to hypotension was not observed. Numerous cases of the use of filtration in adults, children, and animals with septic shock have been reported [170]. However, there are many potential problems with hemofiltration and plasma filtration in sepsis, including vascular access, thromboembolism, mechanical failure, fluid and electrolyte imbalance, and the problems caused by commencing this therapy in unstable patients (i.e., hypotension and hypoxia). Another concern is that this technique removes the inflammatory as well as the anti-inflammatory mediators; these substances cannot be distinguished since they have similar molecular weight [16]. At the present time, the role of filtration in sepsis remains unknown; however, filtration may be considered in septic patients who are ventilated and who receive large doses of inotropes or vasoconstrictors and have a metabolic acidosis or elevated levels of lactate (> 4 mmol/L) [170].

Selective Decontamination of the Digestive Tract (SDD)

SDD targets the potentially pathogenetic gram-negative bacteria in the proximal gastrointestinal tract to avoid colonization of the respiratory system. Therapy typically consists of oral administration of an aminoglycoside, colistin, and amphotericin B. SDD reduced the incidence of respiratory tract colonization and infection, but overall mortality was not affected [288, 289]. Routine clinical use of SDD awaits further supportive evidence.

Corticosteroids

Corticosteroids have been widely used in the past as anti-inflammatory therapy to interrupt the pathophysiologic cascade of events leading to septic shock. However, corticosteroid therapy yielded poor results [290, 291]. Questions regarding the use of corticosteroids in septic shock include the recognition of the patients who will benefit from corticosteroid use, and - for these patients - the dose and the duration of this treatment [292]. Since the 80's, it is generally accepted that corticosteroids should not be used in the management of septic shock. Recent investigators have focused on longer duration therapy with lower doses of corticosteroids [293, 294]. It has been hypothesized that the benefit of corticosteroids may occur with "physiologic" or moderately supraphysiologic doses and that corticosteroids may be most useful for patients with inadequate adrenal reserve, who have persistent shock requiring vasopressors and prolonged mechanical ventilation [292, 295, 296]. Of note, adrenal insufficiency is not uncommon in patients with sepsis and septic shock [297]. Mediators released during sepsis impair synthesis of cortisol via inhibitory actions upon the hypothalamic-pituitary-adrenal axis. Testing involving stimulation by adrenocorticotropin hormones may not be useful in identifying patients with relative adrenal insufficiency. Such patients may have markedly elevated base-line plasma cortisol levels and a blunted response to stimulation by adrenocorticotropic hormones. A random plasma cortisol concentration of less than 20 μg/dl suggests an inadequate adrenal response to stress [298, 299]. Interestingly, in one study, patients who did not have adrenal insufficiency and who received corticosteroids had a slight, albeit not statistically significant, trend toward increased mortality [300]. Other investigators should confirm the finding that low doses of corticosteroids may be beneficial for some septic patients. Clearly, high-dose corticosteroids are contraindicated for the management of patients with sepsis [291].

Nonsteroidal Anti-inflammatory Drugs (NSAIDs)

Nonsteroidal Anti-inflammatory Drugs (NSAIDs) that inhibit cyclo-oxygenase and prostanoid production (such as ibuprofen) reduce the production of metabolites such as thromboxane A_2 (a vasoconstrictor), prostacyclin (a vasodilator), and prostaglandin E_2, which participate in the generation of the clinical presentation of septic shock [301]. However, NSAIDs failed to reduce mortality rate [302].

Drotrecogin Alfa Therapy

Drotrecogin alfa is a recombinant form of human Activated Protein C. It has an anticoagulant action and it is the first anti-inflammatory agent that has proved effective in the treatment of sepsis [303, 304]. Activated protein C inactivates factors Va and VIIIa, thereby preventing the generation of thrombin [304]. Inhibition of thrombin generation by activated protein C decreases inflammation by inhibiting platelet activation, neutrophil recruitment, and mast-cell degranulation. Activated protein C has direct anti-inflammatory properties, including blocking of the production of cytokines by monocytes and blocking cell adhesion [279]. Activated protein C has anti-apoptotic actions that may contribute to its efficacy [305]. The PROWESS trial [303] has demonstrated that the administration of drotrecogin alfa resulted in a 19.4 % reduction in the relative risk of death and an absolute risk reduction of 6.1 % ($p=0.005$). Besides decreasing mortality, activated drotrecogin alfa decreased vasopressor requirements and improved oxygenation in critically ill, septic patients. Patients with APACHE II scores > 25 (i.e., the sicker patients) benefited the most, thus underlying the FDA label that approves drotrecogin alfa (activated) for "severe sepsis and especially for patients at high risk". Effects are less clear for those patients with less severe sepsis. Of note, drotrecogin alfa improved not only short – but also long-term survival [306] and this is an important consideration given that septic patients are at increased risk of death up to 5 years following the septic episode [307].

The major complication associated with drotrecogin alfa (activated) therapy is bleeding; in a recent study, 3.5 % of patients had serious hemorrhage (intracranial hemorrhage, a life-threatening bleeding episode, or a requirement for 3 or more units of blood), as compared with 2 % of patients who received placebo ($p < 0.06$) [308]. Caution is advised in the use of activated protein C in patients with an international normalized ratio (INR) greater than 3 or a platelet count of less than 30.000 / mm^3 [308 - 310]. The role of drotrecogin alfa (activated) in the management of septic patients remains to be determined; despite the relatively good results in some studies, mortality remains high and the costs of this management approach are extremely high [309, 310].

Other Strategies to Restore Defective Anticoagulant Pathways in Sepsis

In addition to a defective protein C system, the other two natural anticoagulant pathways (the antithrombin pathway and tissue factor pathway inhibitor) are incapable of controlling the ongoing thrombin formation [311]. Therapeutic strategies to restore these anticoagulant mechanisms [by the administration of antithrombin concentrates [312, 313], recombinant activated protein C (APC) (see above, drotrecogin therapy), and recombinant TFPI [314, 315] may be a reasonable approach in the supportive treatment of septic patients with coagulation disorders. Experimental and (initial) clinical studies yielded encouraging results not only regarding the reversal of the coagulation disorders, but also regarding organ function and survival [313, 316].

Intensive Insulin Therapy in the ICU

The aim of intensive insulin therapy is to maintain blood glucose levels at 80 – 110 mg / dl by administering insulin. Intensive insulin therapy was associated with an improvement of prognosis of septic patients compared with patients under conventional therapy in which glucose levels ranged between 180 and 200 mg / dl, regardless of whether they had a history of diabetes [317]; first of all, it reduced the frequency of episodes of sepsis by 46 %. It also reduced the overall hospital mortality (by 34 %), and the rate of bloodstream infections by 46 %, acute renal failure requiring dialysis or hemofilration by 41 %, the median number of blood transfusions by 50 %, and critical-illness polyneuropathy by 44 % [317].

The mechanism of this protective action of insulin in septic patients remains unproven. It is well known that hyperglycemia is associated with an impairment of the phagocytic function of neutrophils. Therefore, at least theoretically, restoring glucose levels within normal limits would result in an improvement of bacterial phagocytosis. Moreover, insulin has an antiapoptotic effect, thereby preventing cell death from a variety of stimuli including septic episodes [318]. Given the good results of intensive insulin therapy, it is reasonable to ensure a better control of glucose in critically ill patients by intensive insulin therapy, despite uncertainties about its exact mechanism of action. The disadvantages of intensive insulin therapy is the potential for brain damage secondary to hypoglycemia and the increased staff workload to maintain glucose levels at 80 – 110 mg/dl. An interesting question that should be answered in the future is whether a less tight control of blood glucose – for example a blood glucose level of 120 to 160 mg / dl – provides similar benefits.

Endothelial Cell Replacement

It is well known that the endothelial cells play an active role in the pathophysiology of septic shock; these cells are frequently damaged or die as a result of the septic response, triggering the inflammatory response and aggravating the severity of the situation [319]. Given their role in the development of sepsis, endothelial cell replacement may have in the future a role in the management of critically ill septic patients [320]. Endothelial cell replacement may be achieved through the proliferation of adjacent cells, and – most importantly – by the migration of "progenitor", non-differentiated cells from the bone marrow that adhere to the damaged areas of the microvasculature via the blood circulation.

Antiapoptotic Agents

Increased apoptosis in lymphoid organs and some parenchymal tissues contributes to the immune suppression ("anergy"), and increases the risk of the sepsis-associated MODS / MOFS. Increased apoptosis can be a potential therapeutic target for intervention, particularly by interfering with cell signaling pathways that lead to caspase-mediated apoptosis [321]. In experimental animal studies, strategies that inhibit apoptosis of lymphocytes or gastrointestinal epithelial cells improved survival [322 - 325]. Although clinical trials with anti-apoptotic agents remain distant due in large part to technical difficulties associated with their administration and tissue targeting, inhibition of lymphocytic apoptosis represents an attractive therapeutic target for the septic patient [321, 326].

Advances in the Nutritional Support of Septic Patient

Regarding the nutritional support of the septic patient, current research has focused on methods by which muscle breakdown can be suppressed and accretion of lean body mass can be promoted. Newer approaches have used insulin infusion, growth hormone, IGF-1, IGFBP-3, and proteosome blockers [327 - 329]. Glutamine supplementation also may improve nitrogen balance [330]. The degree of catabolism may be reduced with some of these agents without significant side effects. In addition, they may promote an anabolic response even when calories are provided at levels lower than the resting energy expenditure. This approach ("permissive underfeeding") has been advocated as a means to avoid problems associated with overfeeding (e.g. increased carbon dioxide production, immunosuppression) [331].

Immunomodulation in Sepsis

An impairment of the immune function is common in critically ill septic patients; severe complications and the majority of deaths occur during a prolonged hypoimmune state. Immunomodulation has been proposed in the management of severe sepsis as a means to reverse or prevent immune deficiency [332]. To understand this therapeutic strategy, an in-depth knowledge of the pathophysiology of sepsis – and particularly the alterations of the immune function during the different stages of the evolution of the disease process – is required. During the early phase (hyperinflammatory immune response), anti-inflammatory strategies may result in a significant improvement of outcome [333]. In contrast, anti-inflammatory agents used during the later hypo-immune phase will worsen the prognosis [333, 334]. During this hypo-immune state, agents that stimulate the function of the innate immune system are a reasonable choice [334]. Examples of these immune stimulants include interferon-7 (a potent macrophage activator) [335], interleukin-12 (a potent immune stimulant and Th1 inducer) [336], and antibodies against macrophage migration inhibitory factor [337]. Measurement of circulating concentrations of inflammatory mediators may prove to be useful in evaluating the stage of sepsis and in tailoring the administration of anti-inflammatory agents.

Intravenous administration of immunoglobulins is another alternative in our effort to modulate, in a beneficial manner, the immune response in septic patients [338, 339]. Neutralizing and opsonizing antibodies contained in immunoglobulins may increase serum bactericidal activity, stimulate leukocytes, and neutralize bacterial endo- and exotoxins. IgG and especially IgM antibodies can attenuate cytotoxic effects of complement activation. Furthermore, immunoglobulins can act synergistically with acylureidopenicillins, owing to their content in antilactamase antibodies and their ability to sensitize gram-negative bacteria by disorganizing their outer membranes. Immunoglobulins yielded encouraging results in animal and clinical studies [340, 341]. However, these results were not observed in the whole group of patients with sepsis, but in some particular subgroups, such as patients with postoperative sepsis, septic shock with endotoxemia, neutropenic leukemia patients with sepsis syndrome, children with fulminant meningococcal sepsis, and patients with streptococcal toxic shock syndrome [338]. In these subgroups, serum immunoglobulin levels are often found to be in the lower normal range; the goal of intravenous immunoglobulin administration in these cases is to raise serum levels for at least several days to the upper normal limit or even higher [339, 342]. However, it should be emphasized that other investigators in subsequent larger trials should confirm the results of these studies.

Chapter 6

Monitoring of Shock

Clinical examination for evidence of inadequate tissue perfusion is useful to guide therapy in patients with sepsis. The persistence of fever, leukocytosis, tachycardia, and other findings suggest the presence of active sepsis. Irritability and decreasing conscious state, poor urine output, and poor peripheral perfusion (i.e., rapid, thready pulse and capillary refill > 5 sec) imply inadequate systemic perfusion. Pulse oximetry may suggest hypovolemia and poor perfusion. Body surface temperature measurement is a simple and effective method of assessing the adequacy of tissue perfusion.

Other variables proposed to monitor patients with sepsis, guide therapy, and predict outcome include mean arterial pressure, central venous pressure, Swan-Ganz catheter placement, mixed venous oxygen saturation, oxygen delivery and consumption, gastric mucosal pH value, blood lactate level, and echocardiography [170].

Blood Pressure

Blood pressure monitoring, preferentially by intra-arterial cannulation, is essential. After adequate volume replacement, the systolic and diastolic pressures can be used to guide therapy; a normal or high systolic pressure and a low diastolic pressure imply systemic vasodilation with reasonable ventricular ejection, whereas a low systolic pressure with a high diastolic pressure implies poor ventricular ejection and systemic vasoconstriction.

Central Venous Pressure(CVP)

Central venous catheter placement is essential for patients in septic shock to allow for the infusion of vasoconstrictor drugs and to gain an estimate of left ventricular (LV) end-diastolic volume by measurement of the CVP. CVP can be a poor indicator of volume status in children with pulmonary hypertension, non-compliant right ventricle, poor right ventricular function, tricuspid regurgitation, or pericardial tamponade. A low CVP indicates hypovolemia; however, a normal or high CVP does not rule out hypovolemia.

Swan-Ganz Catheter

Swan-Ganz catheters yield valuable information about a number of significant parameters describing cardiac function (***table 11***). Data gained from pulmonary artery catheter may guide therapy and improve outcome [343].

Table 11. Parameters of cardiac performance

Parameter	Abbreviation	Normal range
Central venous pressure	CVP	1 – 6 mm Hg
Pulmonary Capillary Wedge Pressure	PCWP	6 – 12 mm Hg
Cardiac Index	CI	2.4 – 4.0 L/min/m2
Stroke Volume Index	SVI	40 – 70 mL/beat/m2
Left-Ventricular Stroke Work Index	LVSWI	40 – 60 g.m/m2
Right Ventricle		
Right Ventricular Ejection Fraction	RVEF	40 – 50 %
Right Ventricular End-Diastolic Volume	RVEDV	80 – 150 mL/m2
Right Ventricular Stroke Work Index	RVSWI	4 – 8 g.m/m2
Systemic Vascular Resistance Index	SVRI	1600 – 2400 dynes.sec.m2/cm5
Pulmonary Vascular Resistance Index	PVRI	200 – 400 dynes.sec.m2/cm5

Gastric Intramucosal pH (pHi)

Splanchnic hypoperfusion may be an early sign of systemic hypoperfusion or inadequate resuscitation. pHi measurement is minimally invasive and well tolerated. Newer catheters with a short equilibration time and better measurement techniques will improve the reliability and usefulness of this monitoring method. Over the next few years, pHi measurement has the potential of becoming the gold standard for determining resuscitation and circulatory status in critically ill patients [344, 345].

Serum Lactate Levels

Blood lactate concentration is increased with inadequate perfusion and anaerobic glycolysis. Serum lactate levels can be used to predict outcome in patients with septic shock (***Table 12***) [346, 347]. The upper normal limit of serum lactate is 2 mmol/L. However, in order to have a reasonable prognostic significance, the threshold is defined at 4 mmol/L.

Table 12. Serum lactate levels. Correlation with patient's outcome

	Survivors	**No Survivors**	**Difference**
Cardiac Index (L/min/m2)	3.8	3.9	2.6 %
Oxygen consumption (mL/min/m2)	173	164	5.2 %
Arterial blood lactate (mmol/L)	2.6	7.7	296 %

Measurements in non-survivors were the last before their death
From Ref # 346.

Echocardiography

Transthoracic or transesophageal echocardiography is a non-invasive or minimally invasive, respectively, simple, safe, and repeatable method that provides useful information about myocardial contraction and relaxation (i.e., about systolic and diastolic function; volume status of the patient; presence of a pericardial effusion; and an estimate of pulmonary artery pressure) [348, 349].

Chapter 7

Prognosis and Staging for Sepsis

Prognosis in septic shock depends on many factors. The mortality increases as the severity of the underlying illness increases and in relationship to the predisposing clinical condition [24]. The extremes of age are associated with increased morbidity / mortality in patients with sepsis [350, 351]. Associated co morbidities (neutropenia, chronic diseases, such as cirrhosis, diabetes mellitus, malignancy etc) have a substantial impact on outcome in sepsis modifying both the disease process and the response to therapy [350, 351]. As previously reported (see pathophysiology), genetic factors play a significant role in determining the risk of premature mortality due to sepsis. The outcome of the disease is clearly influenced by other factors, such as the premorbid general health status of the patient, the reversibility of concomitant diseases, and a host of religious and cultural forces that shape the approach toward therapy.

The development of single and multiple organ dysfunction / failure signifies severe sepsis and usually it has a profound effect on the expected morbidity and mortality rate [352 – 354]. The number of failed organs/systems and the duration of the failure adversely affect the prognosis [16]. The average risk of death increases by 15 – 20 % with failure of each additional organ. A median of two organs fails during severe sepsis, with an associated mortality rate of 30 – 40 % [136, 172]. In addition to the number of organ failures, the severity of each failure affects the prognosis. For example, the lower the partial pressure of oxygen, in the case of respiratory failure, and the higher the serum creatinine, in the case of renal failure, the worse the prognosis [166]. The modern organ failure scores can be used to quantitatively describe the degree of organ dysfunction developing over the course of critical illness [355]. However, whether the severity of organ dysfunction can aid in therapeutic stratification is less clear. Fortunately, the majority of organ failures resolve within one month in survivors of sepsis [3]. However, it is interesting to note that septic patients are at increased risk of death up to 5 years following the septic episode [307].

The source of infection is another important determinant of clinical outcome. The greatest risk of developing severe sepsis occurs in the setting of bacteremia associated with nosocomial pneumonia [126]. Patients with intra-abdominal infections and polymicrobial bacteremia or postoperative infections and bacteremia are at significant risk for severe sepsis [126]. Bacteremia associated with intravascular catheters or indwelling urinary catheters carries a lower risk of developing septic shock [357, 358].

The extent of the infection has a significant impact on prognosis. A bilateral bronchopneumonia is a more extensive process than a localized pneumonia, and a generalized fecal peritonitis is a more extensive process than appendicitis.

The type of organism causing the infection is another factor that affects prognosis. The incidence of significant bacteremia is increasing. However, bloodstream invasion is not a prerequisite for the development of septic shock; indeed, only 30 to 50 % of patients with sepsis have positive blood culture results. Gram-positive organisms are responsible for approximately 50 % of bacteremic events [357]. Mortality caused by gram-positive bacteremia has equalled or exceeded death caused by gram-negative bacteremia [357]. Glauser et al [359] found that 57 % of 257 patients with gram-negative sepsis lived, 52 % of 93 patients with gram-positive sepsis lived, 17 % of 9 patients with fungal sepsis lived, and 73 % of 212 patients with no growth on cultures lived. Various pathogens have been identified that increase the risk for shock and death. Bloodstream infection caused by Pseudomonas aeruginosa, Candida albicans, or multidrug resistant Enterococcus faecium is associated with increased mortality [120, 121].

The response of the host to sepsis is another potentially useful prognostic factor. To estimate host response, a number of putative biologic markers of response severity have been used, including circulating levels of procalcitonin [13, 306], IL-6 [361, 362], and others. In addition to their prognostic significance, these biological markers may be used in the process of management decision-making. For example, an indicator of dysregulation of the coagulation system might be more valuable for making a decision about whether to institute therapy with drotrecogin alfa (activated) [303], whereas a marker of adrenal dysfunction might be more useful for determining whether to institute therapy with hydrocortisone [292].

A number of scoring systems have been proposed to assist the clinician in assigning the degree of risk, in assessing the severity of the condition, in quantifying the level of organ dysfunction, and in determining the overall prognosis of the patient with sepsis [363 - 365]. Among the various general outcome prediction models, the most widely used are three: the acute physiology and chronic health evaluation (APACHE) [366, 367], the simplified acute physiology score (SAPS) [365], and the mortality probability models (MPM) [368]. More recently developed scoring systems include the multiple organ dysfunction (MODS) scoring system [18], the sequential organ failure assessment (SOFA) score [354], and the logistic organ dysfunction system (LODS) score [369]. The recently proposed PIRO system (TRIK-5) stratifies patients on the basis of their P (**P**redisposing conditions), the nature and extent of the insult (in the case of sepsis, **I**nfection), the nature and magnitude of the host **R**esponse, and the degree of concomitant **O**rgan dysfunction [4]. The PIRO model needs extensive testing and further refinement in order to be considered ready for routine application in clinical practice. These scoring systems are helpful in the stratification and in the classification of patients for enrolment in clinical trials of new treatments. Moreover, they can be used to describe patient populations in epidemiologic studies for comparison of patients over time or from different institutions. Finally, they may be useful in estimating probabilities of mortality and actual outcomes, which can be compared, creating a standardized mortality ratio (SMR). SMR could then be used to compare ICU performance [370]. However, it should be emphasized that – although these scores are useful in the prediction of mortality of a group of patients – they have not been validated to provide a precise prediction of the outcome of individual patients. Therefore, clinical decisions concerning individual patient care should be taken not only on the basis of any scoring system, but also should be based on clinical assessment and clinical judgment.

Chapter 8

Prevention

Organ dysfunction / failure in the septic patient has a dramatic effect on morbidity and mortality. Given that there is no specific treatment of sepsis-associated MODS/MOFS except organ support, prevention is of particular importance. Therefore, preventive strategies, including optimal vaccine use, effective infection control practices, judicious use and care of intravascular lines and indwelling urinary catheters, use of antibiotic-impregnated central venous catheters, appropriate use of anti-infective agents to prevent microbial resistance, and potentially selective digestive decontamination (see above) should be used to decrease the incidence of infection and subsequent sepsis [119, 236]. Early aggressive enteral nutrition will preserve the integrity of the gastrointestinal epithelium acting as a barrier for the microbes of the intestinal flora, thus preventing microbial translocation [263]. Enteral nutrition may obviate the need for other agents that are used to prevent stress-related gastrointestinal bleeding [16]. Other potential approaches to prevent stress-related gastrointestinal bleeding include the use of histamine type 2 blockers and cytoprotective agents (see above, general supportive measures). As our understanding of the pathophysiology of sepsis progresses, perhaps new modalities will improve clinical outcome.

Another potentially effective method to prevent the development of sepsis is the application of early aggressive therapy in the resuscitation of the septic patient, the so-called "early goal therapy". Early aggressive therapy, that optimizes cardiac preload, after load, and contractility in patients with severe sepsis and septic shock, improves the likelihood of survival [371]. In the study by Rivers et al [371], patients were randomized to receive either standard therapy or early goal-directed therapy before intensive care unit (ICU) transfer and admission. Standard therapy included maintaining a central venous pressure above 8 – 12 mm Hg, the administration of vasopressors for systolic blood pressure less than 90 mm Hg, urine output higher than 0.5 ml/kgr/h, and maintenance of a mean arterial pressure higher than 65 mm Hg. Early goal therapy included the standard approach plus the administration of blood transfusion (red cells, up to an hematocrit of 30 %, to increase oxygen delivery), and the addition of dobutamine when the mixed venous saturation was below 70 %. Resuscitation end points chosen for assessment of the adequacy of oxygen delivery were the normalization of values for mixed venous oxygen saturation, lactate concentration, base deficit, and pH. Patients in the group that received early goal-directed therapy received more fluid, inotropic support, and blood transfusions during the first six hours than did control patients, who received standard resuscitation therapy. During the interval from 7 to 72 hours, patients in the group receiving early goal-directed treatment had a higher mean central venous oxygen concentration, a lower mean lactate concentration, a lower mean base deficit, and a higher mean pH than the control group. Mortality was 30.5 % in the group receiving early goal-directed treatment, as compared with 46.5 % in the control group ($p = 0.009$). Thus, early therapeutic intervention to restore balance between oxygen delivery and oxygen demand improved survival among patients presenting with severe sepsis. The use of objective measures, including lactate concentration, base deficit, pH, and possibly central venous oxygen saturation, in the follow-up of patients who are receiving resuscitation therapy is advisable [279].

Patient screening for genetic variations that may confer susceptibility to sepsis is an approaching reality. A number of genetic polymorphisms (simple gene variations) that may alter the possibility of developing sepsis, including changes in tumor necrosis factors, Toll-like receptors (one of the fundamental bacterial recognition tools in humans), mannose-binding lectin (a primary activator of the complement cascade), and cytokines [29]. Though not a reality today, in the near future it will be possible to rapidly test for such variations on a small scale. However, until we fully understand the intricate and complex role of these polymorphisms, and understand the implications of identifying their variants, we cannot proceed with this most proactive form of sepsis prevention.

Other approaches (such as hormonal manipulations, including administration of gonadal hormones to alter the normal host immune response, and the use of granulocyte-colony stimulating factor to directly influence neutrophil function) in preventing sepsis are currently under investigation.

Chapter 9

Conclusions and Practical Recommendations

Sepsis is an infection-induced syndrome characterized by a generalized inflammatory state. The normal reaction to infection involves a series of complex immunologic processes. A potent, complex immunologic cascade ensures a prompt protective response to microbial invasion in humans. Although activation of the immune system during microbial invasion is generally protective, septic shock develops in a number of patients as a consequence of excessive or poorly regulated immune response to the offending organism. This unbalanced reaction may harm the host through a maladaptive release of endogenously generated inflammatory compounds. Early recognition of the syndrome is of key importance to promptly start appropriate management. Timely, aggressive resuscitation to preserve organ function remains a fundamental principle in the care of septic patients. The specific treatment is directed at identifying and treating the underlying disorder. The physician should investigate diligently for the presence of active infection using modern imaging methods and other diagnostic studies to localize the site of infection and to obtain adequate culture specimens from potential infective sources. Early administration of appropriate, effective antibiotic therapy is important in the management of septic patients. Effective source control is a "Sina Qua Non" in the management of the patient with severe sepsis. Infected fluid collections and / or infected necrotic tissues should be drained or debrided without delay. Adequate nutritional support is indicated in the management of septic patient. A number of adjuvant therapies, aimed at blunting / down-regulating the host immune response to bacterial infection are currently under intensive investigation; however, the complexity of immunologic defenses and the potential for complementary interaction of the different components of the inflammatory cascade make the development of these pharmacological interventions difficult.

References

[1] Sands K, Bates D, Lanken P, et al. Epidemiology of sepsis syndrome in 8 academic medical centers. *JAMA* 1997; 278: 234 – 240.

[2] Parrillo JE, Parker MM, Natanson C, et al. Septic shock in humans. *Ann Intern Med* 1990; 113: 227 – 242.

[3] Wheller AP, Bernard GR. Treating patients with severe sepsis. *N Engl J Med* 1999; 340: 207 – 214.

[4] Levy M, Fink M, Marshall J, et al. 2001 SCCM/ESICM/ACCP/ATS/SIS International Sepsis Definitions Conference. *Crit Care Med* 2003; 31: 1250 – 1256.

[5] Members of the American College of Chest Physicians / Society of Critical Care Medicine Consensus Conference Committee. Definitions for sepsis and organ failure and guidelines for the use of innovative therapies in sepsis. *Crit Care Med* 1992; 20: 864 – 874.

[6] Marshall JC. SIRS and MODS; what is their relevance to the science and practice of intensive care? *Shock* 2000; 14: 586 – 589.

[7] Taniguchi T, Koido Y, Aiboshi J, et al. Change in the ratio of interleukin-6 to interleukin-10 predicts a poor outcome in patients with systemic inflammatory response syndrome. *Crit Care Med* 1999; 27: 1262 – 1264.

[8] Ueda S, Nishio K, Minamino N, et al. Increased plasma levels of adrenomedullin in patients with systemic inflammatory response syndrome. *Am J Respir Crit Care Med* 1999; 160: 132 – 136.

[9] Stoiser B, Knapp S, Thalhammer F, et al. Time course of immunological markers in patients with the systemic inflammatory response syndrome; evaluation of sCD14, sVCAM-1, sELAM, MIP-1 alpha and TGF-beta2. *Eur J Clin Invest* 1998; 28: 672 – 678.

[10] Hietaranta A, Kemppainen E, Puolakkainen P, et al. Extracellular phospholipases A_2 in relation to systemic inflammatory response syndrome (SIRS) and systemic complications in severe acute pancreatitis. *Pancreas* 2002; 18: 385 – 391.

[11] Takala A, Jousela I, Olkkola KT, et al. Systemic inflammatory response syndrome without systemic inflammation in acutely ill patients admitted to hospital in a medical emergency. *Clin Sci* 1999; 96: 287 – 295.

[12] Sablotzki A, Borgermann J, Baulig W, et al. Lipopolysaccharide-binding protein (LBP) and markers of acute-phase response in patients with multiple organ dysfunction syndrome (MODS) following open heart surgery. *Thorac Cardiovasc Surg* 2001; 49: 273 – 278.

[13] Harbarth S, Holeckova K, Froidevaux C, et al. Diagnostic value of procalcitonin, interleukin-6, and interleukin-8 in critically ill patients admitted with suspected sepsis. *Am J Respir Crit Care Med* 2001; 164: 396 – 340.

[14] Duflo F, Debon R, Monneret G, et al. Alveolar and serum procalcitonin: Diagnostic and prognostic value in ventilator-associated pneumonia. *Anesthesiology* 2002; 96: 74 – 79.

[15] Matuschak GM. Multiple systems organ failure; clinical expression, pathogenesis, and therapy. In: Hall JB, Schmidt GA, Wood LDH (Eds) *Principles of Critical Care*, McGraw-Hill Inc Ed, New York, 1992, pp 613 – 636.

[16] Balk RA. Pathogenesis and management of multiple organ dysfunction or failure in severe sepsis and septic shock. *Crit Care Clin* 2000; 16: 337 – 352.

[17] Angus DC, Linde-Zwirble WT, Lidicer J, et al. Epidemiology of severe sepsis in the United States: analysis of incidence, outcome, and associated costs of care. *Crit Care Med* 2001; 29: 1303 – 1310.

[18] Marshall JC, Cook DJ, Christou NV, et al. Multiple organ dysfunction score: a reliable descriptor of a complex clinical outcome. *Crit Care Med* 1995; 23: 1638 – 1652.

[19] Ferreira FL, Bota DP, Bross A, et al. Serial evaluation of the SOFA score to predict outcome in critically ill patients. *JAMA* 2002; 286: 1754-1758.

[20] Wilkinson JD, Pollack MM, Ruttiman M, et al. Outcome of pediatric patient with multiple organ system failure. *Crit Care Med* 1986; 14: 271-274.

[21] Proulx F, Fagan M, Farrell CA, et al. Epidemiology of sepsis and multiple organ dysfunction syndrome in children. *Chest* 1996; 109: 1033-1037.

[22] Doughty LA, Carcillo JA, Kaplan SS, et al. Plasma nitrite and nitrate concentration and multiple organ failure in pediatric sepsis. *Crit Care Med* 1996; 109: 1033-1037.

[23] Carcillo JA, Task Force Members, Fields AI. Clinical practice parameters for hemodynamic support of pediatrics and neonatal patients in septic shock. *Crit Care Med* 2002; 30: 1 – 13.

[24] Balk RA. Severe sepsis and septic shock. Definitions, epidemiology, and clinical manifestations. *Crit Care Clin* 2000; 16: 179 – 192.

[25] Center for Disease Control (CDC). Increase in national hospital discharge survey for septicemia – United States 1979 – 1987. *Morbid Mortal Weekly Rep* 1990; 39: 31 – 34.

[26] Richards MJ, Edwards JR, Culver DH, et al. Nosocomial infections in medical intensive care units in the United States. *Crit Care Med* 1999; 27: 887 – 892.

[27] Martin GS, Mannino DM, Moss IM. Sepsis trends in the United States. *Crit Care Med* 2001; 29: A8.

[28] Martin GS. Research into sepsis pathophysiology unlocks potential future therapies. *http://www.medscape.com/viewarticle/455752* (2003).

[29] Mira J-P. *Clinical sepsis: genetic predisposition*. Program and abstracts of the 23rd International Symposium on Intensive Care and Emergency Medicine; March 18 – 21, 2003; Brussels, Belgium.

[30] Rangel-Frausto MS, Pittet D, Costigan M, et al. The natural history of the systemic inflammatory response syndrome (SIRS). A prospective study. *JAMA* 1995; 273: 117 – 123.

[31] Rangel – Frausto M. The epidemiology of bacterial sepsis. *Infect Dis Clin North Am* 1999; 13: 299 – 312.

[32] Brun-Buisson C, Doyon F, Carlet J, et al. Incidence, risk factors, and outcome of severe sepsis and septic shock in adults: a multicenter prospective study in intensive care units. JAMA 1995; 274: 968 – 974.

[33] Kieft H, Hoepelman AI, Zhou W, et al. The sepsis syndrome in a Dutch university hospital. Clinical observations. *Arch Intern Med* 1993; 153: 2241 – 2247.

[34] Hardaway RM. A review of septic shock. *Am Surg* 2000; 66:22 – 29.

[35] Rodrigues JC, Fein AM. Diagnostic approach and clinical manifestations of severe sepsis. In: Fein AM, Abraham EM, Balk RA, et al (Eds) *Sepsis and Multiorgan Failure*. Baltimore, Williams & Wilkins, 1997, pp 269 – 276.

[36] Kieft H. *The sepsis syndrome. Clinical observations, microbiologic features, new treatment modalities*. Utrecth, the Netherlands, University of Utrecht, 1994, Thesis, pp 104.

[37] Baker CC, Huynh T. Sepsis in the critically ill patient. *Curr Probl Surg* 1995; 32: 1013 – 1092.

[38] Hack CE, Nuijens JH, Strack van Schijndel RI, et al. A model for the interplay of inflammatory mediators in sepsis – a study in 48 patients. *Intensive Care Med* 1990; 16 (Suppl 3): S187 – S191.

[39] Fearon DT, Locksley RM. The instructive role of innate immunity in the acquired immune response. *Science* 1996; 272: 50 – 53.

[40] Hack CE, Zeerleder S. The endothelium in sepsis: Source of and a target for inflammation. *Crit Care Med* 2001; 29 (Suppl): S21 – S27.

[41] Mileski WJ. Sepsis. What it is and how to recognize it. *Surg Clin North Am* 1991; 71: 749 – 764.

[42] Unanue ER, Allen PM. The basis for the immunoregulatory role of macrophages and other accessory cells. *Science* 1987; 236: 551 – 557.

[43] Border JR. Multiple systems organ failure. *Ann Surg* 1992; 216: 111 – 116.

[44] Deitch EA. Multiple organ failure: pathophysiology and potential future therapy. *Ann Surg* 1992; 216: 117 – 134.

[45] Weiss S. Tissue destruction by neutrophils. *N Engl J Med* 1989; 320: 365 – 376.

[46] Goya T, Morisaki T, Torisu M. Immunologic assessment of host defense impairment in patients with septic multiple organ failure: relationship between complement activation and changes in neutrophil function. *Surgery* 1994; 115: 145 – 155.

[47] Simms HH, D' Amico R. Polymicrobial sepsis disrupts normal neutrophil extracellular matrix protein interactions. *Shock* 1992; 38: 1 – 8.

[48] Muller MM, Griesmacher A. Markers of endothelial dysfunction. *Clin Chem Lab Med* 2000; 38: 77 – 85.

[49] Pober JS, Cotran RS. Cytokines and endothelial cell biology. *Physiol Rev* 1990; 70: 427 – 451.

[50] Vane JR, Anggard EE, Botting RM. Regulatory functions of the vascular endothelium. *N Engl J Med* 1990; 323: 27 – 36.

[51] Osborne L. Leukocyte adhesion to endothelium in inflammation. *Cell* 1990; 62: 3 – 6.

[52] Douzinas EE, Tsismetziadou PD, Pitardis MT, et al. The regional production of cytokines and lactate in sepsis-related multiple organ failure. *Am J Respir Crit Care Med* 1997; 155: 53 – 59.

[53] Cotran RS. New roles for the endothelium in inflammation and immunity. *Am J Pathol* 1987; 129: 407 – 413.

[54] Casey LC. Immunologic response to infection and its role in septic shock. *Crit Care Clin* 2000; 16: 193 – 213.

[55] Christman JW, Wheller AP, Bernard GR. Cytokines and sepsis: what are the therapeutic implications? *J Intensive Care* 1991; 6: 172 – 182.

[56] Strieter RM, Kunkel SL. Acute lung injury: the role of cytokines in the elicitation of neutrophils. *J Invest Med* 1994; 42: 640 – 651.

[57] Carlos TM, Harlan JM. Leukocyte-endothelial adhesion molecules. *Blood* 1994; 84: 2068 – 2101.

[58] Sessler CN, Windsor AC, Schwartz M, et al. Circulating ICAM-1 is increased in septic shock. *Am J Respir Crit Care Med* 1995; 151: 1420 – 1427.

[59] van der Poll T, Buller HR, ten Cate H, et al. Activation of coagulation after administration of tumor necrosis factor to normal subjects. *N Engl J Med* 1990; 322: 1622 – 1627.

[60] Beutler B, Cerami A. Cachectin: more than a tumor necrosis factor. *N Engl J Med* 1987; 316: 379 – 385.

[61] Tracey KJ, Beutler B, Lowry SF, et al. Shock and tissue injury induced by recombinant human cachectin. *Science* 1986; 234: 470 – 474.

[62] Dinarello C. The inflammatory cytokines interleukin-1, tumor necrosis factor and treatment of septic shock. *J Infect Dis* 1991; 163: 1177 – 1184.

[63] Waage A, Halstensen A, Espevic T. Association between tumor necrosis factor in serum and fatal outcome in patients with meningococcal disease. *Lancet* 1987; 1: 355 – 377.

[64] Herbertson MJ, Werner HA, Goddard CM, et al. Anti-tumor necrosis factor-alpha prevents decreased ventricular contractility in endotoxemic pigs. *Am J Respir Crit Care Med* 1995; 152: 480 – 488.

[65] Schag G, Redl H, Davies J, Haller I. Anti-tumor necrosis factor antibody treatment of recurrent bacteremia in a baboon model. *Shock* 1994; 2: 10 – 18.

[66] Okusow S, Gelfand JA, Ikejima T, et al. Interleukin-1 induces a shock-like state in rabbits. Synergism with tumor necrosis factor and the effect of cyclooxygenase inhibitors. *J Clin Invest* 1988; 81: 1162 – 1172.

[67] Light RB. Sepsis syndrome. In: Hall JB, Schmidt GA, Wood LDH (Eds) *Principles of Critical Care*, McGraw-Hill Inc Ed, New York, 1992, pp 645 - 655.

[68] Casey LC, Balk RA, Bone RC. Plasma cytokine and endotoxin levels correlate with survival in patients with sepsis syndrome. *Ann Intern Med* 1993; 119: 771 – 778.

[69] Wakabayaski G, Gelfand JA, Burke JF, et al. A specific receptor antagonist for inteleukin-1 prevents Escherichia coli – induced shock in rabbits. *FASEB J* 1991; 5: 338 – 343.

[70] Fisher CJ, Stolman GJ, Opal SM, et al. Initial evaluation of human recombinant interleukin-1 receptor antagonist in the treatment of sepsis syndrome. The IL-1ra Sepsis Syndrome Study Group. *Crit Care Med* 1994; 22: 12 – 21.

[71] Baggiolini M, Dewald B, Moser B. Interleukin-8 and related chemotactic cytokines. *Adv Immunol* 1994; 55: 97 – 179.

[72] Marty C, Misset B, Tamion F, et al. Circulating interleukin-8 concentrations in patients with multiple organ failure of septic and non-septic origin. *Crit Care Med* 1994; 22: 673 – 679.

[73] Zee KJ, De Foege LE, Fischer E, et al. IL-8 in septic shock, endotoxemia, and after IL-1 administration. *J Immunol* 1991; 146: 3478 – 3482.

[74] Howard M, Muchamel T, Andrade S. Interleukin 10 protects mice from lethal endotoxemia. *J Exper Med* 1993; 177: 1205 – 1208.

[75] Friedman G, Jankowski S, Marchant A, et al. Blood interleukin 10 levels parallel the severity of septic shock. *J Crit Care* 1997; 12: 183 – 187.

[76] Gomez-Jimenez J, Martin MC, Sauri R, et al. Interleukin 10 and the monocyte / macrophage-induced inflammatory response in septic shock. *J Infect Dis* 1995; 171: 472 – 475.

[77] Sakorafas GH, Tsiotos GG, Sarr MG. Ischemia / reperfusion induced pancreatitis. *Dig Surg* 2000; 17: 3 – 14.

[78] Lowenstein CJ, Dinermal JL, Snyder SH. Nitric oxide: a physiologic messenger. *Ann Intern Med* 1994; 120: 227 – 237.

[79] Lancaster Jr JR. Nitric oxide in cells. *Am Sci* 1992; 80: 248 – 259.

[80] Vedas P. Elevated plasma PLA_2: correlation with the hemodynamic and pulmonary changes in Gram-negative septic shock. *J Lab Clin Med* 1984; 104: 873 – 881.

[81] Vedas P, Pruzanskiw H, Stefanski E, et al. Pathogenesis of hypotension in septic shock: correlation of circulatory PLA_2 levels with circulatory collapse. *Crit Care Med* 1988; 16: 1 – 10.

[82] Anderson BO, Bensard DD, Harken AH. The role of PAF and its antagonists in shock, sepsis, and multiple organ failure. *Surg Gynecol Obstet* 1991; 172: 415 – 424.

[83] Chao W, Olson MS. Platelet-activating factor: receptors and signal transduction. *Biochem J* 1993; 292: 617 – 629.

[84] Petrak RA, Balk RA, Bone RC. Prostaglandins, cyclo-oxygenase inhibitors, and thromboxane synthesis inhibitors in the pathogenesis of multiple organ failure. *Crit Care Clin* 1989; 5: 303 – 314.

[85] Bone RC. Phospholipids and their inhibitors: a critical evaluation of their role in the treatment of sepsis. *Crit Care Med* 1992; 20: 884 – 890.

[86] Taylor F, Levi M, Artigas A, et al. Sepsis: Inflammation disorder, coagulation disorder, or both? A challenge for clinicians. *Crit Care Med* 2001; 29 (Suppl): S 107 – S109.

[87] Marshall JC. Inflammation, coagulopathy, and the pathogenesis of multiple organ dysfunction syndrome. *Crit Care Med* 2001; 29 (Suppl): S 99 – S106.

[88] Dosquet C, Weill D, Wautier JL. Cytokines and thrombosis. *J Cardiovasc Pharmacol* 1995; 25 (Suppl 2): S13 – S19.

[89] Fourrier F, Chopin C, Goudemand J, et al. Septic shock, multiple organ failure, and disseminated intravascular coagulation. *Chest* 1992; 101: 816 – 823.

[90] Cate H. Pathophysiology of disseminated intravascular coagulation in sepsis. *Crit Care Med* 2000; 28 (Suppl): S9 – S11.

[91] Dorinsky PM, Gadek JE. Mechanism of multiple nonpulmonary organ failure in ARDS. *Chest* 1989; 96: 885 – 892.

[92] Kirschfink M. Controlling the complement system in inflammation. *Immunopharmacology* 1997; 38: 51-62.

[93] Hangen DH, Stevens JH, Satoh PS, et al. Complement levels in septic primates treated with anti-C5a antibodies. *J Surg Res* 1989; 46: 195 – 199.

[94] Saadia R, Schein M, Mac Farlane C, et al. Gut barrier function and the surgeon. *Br J Surg* 1990; 77: 487 – 492.

[95] Swank GM, Deitch EA. Role of the gut in multiple organ failure: Bacterial translocation and permeability changes. *World J Surg* 1996; 20: 411 – 417.

[96] Baue AE. The role of the gut in the development of multiple organ dysfunction in cardiothoracic patients. *Ann Thorac Surg* 1993; 55: 822 – 829.

[97] Crouser ED, Dorinsky PM. Gastrointestinal tract dysfunction in critical illness: Pathophysiology and interaction with acute lung injury in adult respiratory distress syndrome / multiple organ dysfunction syndrome. *New Orizons* 1994; 2: 476 – 487.

[98] Dhainaut J-F, Marin N, Mignon A, Vinsonneau C. Hepatic response to sepsis: Interaction between coagulation and inflammatory process. *Crit Care Med* 2001; 29 (Suppl): S42 – S47.

[99] Doi F, Goya T, Torisu M. Potential role of hepatic macrophages in neutrophil-mediated liver injury in rats with sepsis. *Hepatology* 1993; 17: 1086 – 1094.

[100] Abel FL. Myocardial function in sepsis and endotoxin shock. *Am J Physiol* 1989; 57: 1265 – 1281.

[101] Kumar A, Haery C, Parrillo JE. Myocardial dysfunction in septic shock. *Crit Care Clin* 2000; 16: 251 – 288.

[102] Parker MM, McCarthy KE, Ognibene FP, Parillo JE. Right ventricular dysfunction and dilatation, similar to left ventricular changes, characterize the cardiac depression of septic shock in humans. *Chest* 1990; 97: 126 – 131.

[103] Oberholzer K, Oberhoizer A, Clare-Salzeer M, Moldawer LL. Apoptosis in sepsis: a new target for therapeutic exploration. *FASEB J* 2001; 15: 879 – 892.

[104] Berczi I. Neuroendocrine response to endotoxin. *Ann N Y Acad Sci* 1998; 851: 411 – 415.

[105] Berczi I. Neurohormonal host defense in endotoxin shock. *Ann N Y Acad Sci* 1998; 840: 787 – 802.

[106] Bolton CF. Sepsis and the systemic inflammatory response syndrome: Neuromuscular manifestations. *Crit Care Med* 1996; 24: 1408 – 1416.

[107] McIntyre L, Walley KR. Importance of underlying mechanism and genotype on outcome of sepsis trials. *Crit Care Med* 2001; 29: 677 – 679.

[108] Kumar A, Short J, Parillo JE. Genetic factors in septic shock. *JAMA* 1999; 282: 579 – 581.

[109] Mira JP, Cariou A, Grall F, et al. Association of TNF_2, a TNF-alpha promoter polymorphism, with septic shock susceptibility and mortality: A multicenter study, *JAMA* 1999; 282: 561 – 568.

[110] Fang XM, Schroder S, Hoeft A, et al. Comparison of two polymorphisms of the IL-1 gene family: IL-1 receptor antagonist polymorphism contributes to susceptibility to severe sepsis. *Crit Care Med* 1999; 27: 1330 – 1334.

[111] Barton R, Cerra FB. The hypermetabolism: Multiple organ failure syndrome. *Chest* 1989; 96: 1153 – 1160.

[112] Mizock BA. Metabolic derangements in sepsis and septic shock. *Crit Care Clin* 2000; 16: 319 – 336.

[113] Fink M. Cytopathic hypoxia in sepsis. *Acta Anaesth Scand* 1997; 110 (Suppl): 87 – 115.

[114] Kreger BE, Craven DE, Carling PC, et al. Gram-negative bacteremia III. Reassessment of etiology, epidemiology, and ecology in 612 patients. *Am J Med* 1980; 68: 332 – 343.

[115] Brun-Buisson C, Doyon F, Carlet J, et al. Bacteremia and severe sepsis in adults: A multicenter prospective survey in ICUs and wards of 24 hospitals. *Am J Respir Crit Care Med* 1996; 154: 617 – 623.

[116] Bernal A, Proft T, Fraser JD. Superantigens in human disease. *J Clin Immunol* 1999; 19: 149 – 157.

[117] Bannan J, Visvanathan K, Zabriskie JB. Structure and function of streptococcal and staphylococcal superantigens in septic shock. *Infect Dis Clin North am* 1999; 13: 387 – 396.

[118] Geerdes H, Ziegler D, Lode H, et al. Septicemia in 980 patients at a university hospital in Berlin: Prospective studies during 4 selected years between 1979 and 1989. *Clin Infect Dis* 1992; 15: 991 – 998.

[119] Simon D, Trenholme G. Antibiotic selection for patients with septic shock. *Crit Care Clin* 2000; 16: 215 – 231.

[120] Linden P, Pasculle A, Manez R, et al. Differences in outcomes for patients with bacteremia due to Vancomycin-resistant Enterococcus faecium or Vancomycin – susceptible E. faecium. *Clin Infect Dis* 1996; 22: 663 – 668.

[121] Miller P, Wenzel R. Etiologic organisms as independent predictors of death and morbidity associated with bloodstream infections. *J Infect Dis* 1987; 156: 471 – 478.

[122] Wenzel R. Nosocomial candidemia: Risk factors and attributable mortality. *Clin Infect Dis* 1995; 20: 1531 – 1538.

[123] Darby JM, Linden P, Pasculle W, Saul M. Utilization and diagnostic yield of blood cultures in a surgical intensive care unit. *Crit Care Med* 1997; 25: 989 – 994.

[124] O' Grady NP, Barie PS, Bartlett JG, et al. Practice guidelines for evaluating new fever in critically ill adult patients. Task Force of the Society of Critical Care Medicine and the Infectious Diseases Society of America. *Clin Infect Dis* 1998; 26: 1042 – 1059.

[125] Gleckman R, Hibert D. Afebrile bacteremia: a phenomenon in geriatric patients. *JAMA* 1982; 248: 1478 – 1481.

[126] Llewelyn M, Cohen J. Diagnosis of infection in sepsis. *Intensive Care Med* 2001; 27: S10 – S32.

[127] Carlet J. Rapid diagnostic methods in the detection of sepsis. *Infect Dis Clin North Am* 1999; 13: 483 – 494.

[128] Yentis SM, Soni N, Sheldon J. C-reactive protein as an indicator of resolution of sepsis in the intensive care unit. *Intensive Care Med* 1995; 21: 602 – 605.

[129] Oberhoffer M, Karzai W, Meier-Hellmann A, et al. Sensitivity and specificity of various markers of inflammation for the prediction of tumor necrosis factor-alpha and interleukin-6 in patients with sepsis. *Crit Care Med* 1999; 27: 1814 – 1818.

[130] Ugarte H, Silva E, Mercan D, et al. Procalcitonin used as a marker of infection in the intensive care unit. *Crit Care Med* 1999; 27: 498 – 504.

[131] Whang KT, Steinwald PM, White JC, et al. Serum calcitonin precursors in sepsis and systemic inflammation. *J Clin Endocrinol Metab* 1998; 83: 3296 – 3301.

[132] Povoa P, Almeida E, Moreira P, et al. C-reactive protein as an indicator of sepsis. *Intensive Care Med* 1998; 24: 1052 – 1056.

[133] de Werra I, Jaccard C, Corradin SB, et al. Cytokines, nitrite/nitrate, soluble tumor necrosis factor receptors, and procalcitonin concentrations: comparisons in patients with septic shock, cardiogenic shock, and bacterial pneumonia. *Crit Care Med* 1997; 25: 607 – 613.

[134] Hatherill M, Tibby S, Sykes T, et al. Diagnostic markers of infection: comparison of procalcitonin with C reactive protein and leucocyte count. *Arch Dis Child* 1999; 81: 417 – 421.

[135] Sakorafas GH. *Multiple organ failure syndrome*. Monograph, Athens 1990, Diaton Ed, pp 50.

[136] Hebert PC, Drummond AJ, Singer J, Bernard GR, Russell JA. A simple multiple system organ failure scoring system predicts mortality of patients who have sepsis syndrome. *Chest* 1993; 104: 230 – 235.

[137] Piper RD, Sibbald WJ. Multiple organ dysfunction syndrome: The relevance of persistent infection and inflammation. In: Fein AM, Abraham ED, Balk RA, et al (Eds). *Sepsis and multiorgan failure*. Baltimore, Williams & Wilkins, 1997, pp 189 – 208.

[138] Light RB. Septic shock. In: Hall JB, Schmidt GA, Wood LDH (Eds) *Principles of critical care*, New York, McGraw-Hill, 1992, pp 1172 – 1185.

[139] Field S, Kelly SM, Macklem PT. The oxygen cost of breathing with cardiorespiratory disease. *Am Rev Respir Dis* 1982; 126: 9 – 13.

[140] Martin GS, Bernard GR. Airway and lung in sepsis. *Intensive Care Med* 2001; 27: S63 – S79.

[141] Tobin MJ. Mechanical ventilation. *N Engl J Med* 1994; 330: 1056 – 1061.

[142] Stoller JK. Current controversies in applying specific modes of mechanical ventilation. In: Hall JB, Schmidt GA, Wood LDH (Eds) *Principles of critical care*, New York, McGraw-Hill, 1992, pp 155 - 159.

[143] Carmichael LC, Dormisky PM, Higgins SB, et al. Diagnosis and therapy of acute respiratory distress syndrome in adults: an international survey. *J Crit Care* 1996; 11: 9 – 18.

[144] Hickling KG. Permissive hypercapnia. *Respir Care Clin North Am*. 2002; 8: 155 - 169.

[145] McHugh LG, Milberg JA, Whitcomb ME, et al. Recovery of function in survivors of the acute respiratory distress syndrome. *Am J Respir Crit Care Med* 1994; 150: 90 – 94.

[146] Hall JB, Wood LDH. Liberation of the patient from mechanical ventilation. *JAMA* 1987; 257: 1621 – 1627.

[147] Bone RC. Sepsis syndrome; new insights into its pathogenesis and treatment. *Infect Dis Clin North Am* 1991; 5: 793 – 805.

[148] Pulmonary artery catheter consensus conference: consensus statement. *Crit Care Med* 1997; 25: 910 – 925.

[149] Connors AF Jr, Speroff T, Dawson NV, et al. The effectiveness of right heart catheterization in the initial care of critically ill patients. *JAMA* 1996; 276: 889 – 897.

[150] Abou-Khalil B, Scalea TM, Trooskin SZ, Henry SM, Hitchcock R. Hemodynamic responses to shock in young trauma patients: need for intensive monitoring. *Crit Care Med* 1994; 22: 633 – 639.

[151] Vincent JL. Hemodynamic support in septic shock. *Intensive Care Med* 2001; 27: S80 – S92.

[152] Rackow EC, Falk JL, Fein IA, et al. Fluid resuscitation in septic shock. *Crit Care Med* 1983; 11: 839 – 850.

[153] Meumann M, Demling RH. Colloid vs. crystalloid: a current perspective. *Confed Aust Crit Care Nurses J*; 1990; 3: 30 – 35.

[154] Levine R, Alvarez FG. Intravenous fluid therapy. *Hosp Physician* 1994; 30: 21 – 37.

[155] Velanovich V. Crystalloid versus colloid fluid resuscitation: meta-analysis of mortality. *Surgery* 1989; 105: 65 – 71.

[156] Bunnell E, Parrillo JE. Cardiac dysfunction during septic shock. *Clin Chest Med* 1996; 17: 237 – 248.

[157] Walley KR, Wood LDH. Cardiovascular disorders in the critically ill . In Hall JB, Schmidt GA, Wood LDH (Eds) *Principles of Critical Care*, McGraw-Hill (ed), New York, 1992, pp 1393 – 1416.

[158] Hayes MA, Yau EHS, Timmins AC, Hinds CJ, Watson D. Response of the critically ill patients to treatment aimed at achieving supranormal oxygen delivery and consumption. *Chest* 1993; 103: 886 – 895.

[159] Cooper DJ, Walley KR, Wiggs BR, Russell JA. Bicarbonate does not improve hemodynamics in critically ill patients who have lactic acidosis: a prospective, controlled clinical study. *Ann Intern Med* 1990; 112: 492 – 498.

[160] Boyd O, Grounds M, Bennett ED. A randomized clinical trial of the effect of deliberate perioperative increase of oxygen delivery on mortality in high-risk surgical patients. *JAMA* 1993; 270: 2699 – 2707.

[161] Russell JA, Phang PT. The oxygen delivery / consumption controversy: approaches to management of the critically ill. *Am J Respir Crit Care Med* 1995; 149: 533 – 537.

[162] Gattinoni L, Brazzi L, Pelosi P, et al. A trial of goal-oriented hemodynamic therapy in critically ill patients. *N Engl J Med* 1995; 333: 1025 – 1032.

[163] Hebert PC, Wells G, Blajchman MA, et al. A multicenter, randomized, controlled clinical trial of transfusion requirements in critical care. *N Engl J Med* 1999; 340: 409 – 417.

[164] Hayes MA, Timmins AC, Yau EH, Palazzo M, Hinds CJ, Watson D. Elevation of systemic oxygen delivery in the treatment of critically ill patients. *N Engl J Med* 1994; 330: 1717 - 1722.

[165] Marik PE, Sibbald WI. Effect of stored-blood transfusion on oxygen delivery in patients with sepsis. *JAMA* 1993; 269: 3044 – 3029.

[166] Wheeler A, Carmichael L, Christman B, et al. Renal function abnormalities in sepsis. *Am J Respir Crit Care Med* 1995; 151 (Suppl) A317.

[167] Marini JJ, Wright L. General supportive care of the critically ill patient. *Semin Respir Crit Care Med* 1997; 18: 3 – 17.

[168] Cook D. Prevention of stress ulcers and ventilator-associated pneumonia. *Semin Respir Crit Care Med* 1997; 18: 91 – 95.

[169] Jain M, Schmidt GA. Venous thromboembolism: prevention and prophylaxis. *Semin Respir Crit Care Med* 1997; 18: 79 – 90.

[170] Butt W. Septic shock. *Pediatr Clin North Am* 2001; 48: 601 – 625.

[171] Carcillo JA. Pediatric septic shock and multiple organ failure. *Crit Care Clin* 2003; 19: 413-40, viii.

[172] Pittet D, Thievent B, Wenzel RP, et al. Bedside prediction of mortality from bacteremic sepsis: a dynamic analysis of ICU patients. *Am J Respir Crit Care Med* 1996; 153: 684 – 693.

[173] Stone HH, Bourneuf AA, Stinson LD. Reliability of criteria for predicting persistent or recurrent sepsis. *Arch Surg* 1985; 120: 17 – 20.

[174] Gold H, Moellering R. Antimicrobial-drug resistance. *N Engl J Med* 1996; 335: 1445 – 1448.

[175] Smith T, Pearson M, Wilcox K, et al. Emergence of vancomycin resistance in Staphylococcal aureus. *N Engl J Med* 1999; 340: 493 – 498.

[176] Friedland I, McCracken G. Management of infections caused by antibiotic-resistant Streptococcus pneumoniae. *N Engl J Med* 1994; 331: 377 – 381.

[177] Chen D, McGeer A, de Azavedo J, Low DE. Decreased susceptibility of Streptococcus pneumoniae to fluoroquinolones in Canada. *N Engl J Med* 1999; 341: 233 – 238.

[178] Craig WA. Qualitative susceptibility tests versus quantitative MIC tests. *Diagn Microbiol Infect Dis* 1993; 16: 231 – 236.

[179] Hurley JC. Antibiotic – induced release of endotoxin: a reappraisal. *Clin Infect Dis* 1992; 15: 84 – 92.

[180] Jenkins JK, Carey PD., Byrne K, Sugerman HJ, Fowler AA 3rd. Sepsis-induced lung injury and effects of ibuprofen pretreatment: analysis of early alveolar events via repetitive bronchoalveolar lavage. *Am Rev Respir Dis* 1991; 143: 155 – 161.

[181] Stillwell M, Caplan ES. The septic multiple trauma patient. *Infect Dis Clin North Am* 1989; 3: 155 – 183.

[182] Bohnen JM, Solomkin JS, Dellinger PE, Bjornson HS, Page CP. Guidelines for clinical care; anti-infection agents for intra-abdominal infection. A Surgical Infection Society policy statement. *Arch Surg* 1992; 127: 83 – 89.

[183] Jimenez MF, Marshall JC. Source control in the management of sepsis. *Intensive Care Med* 2001; 27: S49 – S62.

[184] Sprung CL, Finch RG, Thijs LG, Glauser MP. International sepsis trial (INTERSEPT): role and impact of a clinical evaluation committee. *Crit Care Med* 1996; 24: 1441 -1447.

[185] Sakorafas GH. Multi-organ failure as an indication for exploratory laparotomy. *Arch Hellenic Surg* (Gr) 1989, 56: 37 - 42.

[186] Kaul R, McGeer A, Low DE, Green K, Schwartz B. Population-based surveillance for group A streptococcal necrotizing fasciitis: clinical features, prognostic indicators, and microbiological analysis of seventy-seven cases. Ontario Group A Streptococcal study. *Am J Med* 1997; 103: 18 – 24.

[187] Eriksson B, Andersson J, Holm SE, Norgren M. Epidemiological and clinical aspects of invasive group A streptococcal infection and the streptococcal toxic shock syndrome. *Clin Infect Dis* 1998; 27: 1428 – 1436.

[188] Majeski JA, Alexander JW. Early diagnosis and surgical treatment of necrotizing fasciitis. *Surg Gynecol Obstet* 1983; 157: 784 – 200.

[189] Moss RL, Musemeche CA, Kosloske AM. Necrotizing fasciitis in children: prompt recognition and aggressive therapy improve survival. *J Pediatr Surg* 1996; 31: 1142 – 1146.

[190] Adant JP, Bluth F, Fissetter J. Necrotizing fasciitis; a life-threatening infection. *Acta Chir Belg* 1998; 98: 102 – 106.

[191] Condon RE. Necrotizing skin and soft tissue infections. In: *Conn's current therapy*. Rakel R, Ed. WB Saunders ED, Philadelphia, 1998, pp 87 – 90.

[192] Bilton BD, Zibari GB, McMillan RW, Aultman DF, Dunn G, McDonald JC. Aggressive surgical management of necrotizing fasciitis serves to decrease mortality; a retrospective study. *Am Surg* 1998; 64: 397 – 400.

[193] Lewis RT. Soft tissue infections. *World J Surg* 1998; 22: 146 – 155.

[194] Brown G, Chamberlain R, Goulding J, Clarke A. Ceftriaxone versus cefazolin with probenecid for severe skin and soft tissue infections. *J Emerg Med* 1996; 14: 547 – 551.

[195] McHenry CR, Brandt CP, Piotrowski JJ, Jacobs DG, Malagnoni MA. Idiopathic necrotizing fasciitis; recognition, incidence, and outcome of therapy. *Am Surg* 1994; 60: 490 – 494.

[196] Davies HD, McGeer A, Schartz B, et al. The Ontario Group A Streptococcal Study Group. Invasive group A streptococcal infections in Ontario, Canada. *N Engl J Med* 1996; 335: 547 – 554.

[197] Nichols RL. Diagnosis and treatment of uncomplicated and complicated surgical infections. *Surgery* 2000; 128: S19 – S30.

[198] Laor E, Palmer LS, Tolia BM, Reid RE, Winter HI. Outcome prediction in patients with Fournier's gangrene. *J Urol* 1995; 154: 89 – 92.

[199] Bartlet P, Reingold AL, Graham DR, et al. Toxic shock associated with surgical wound infection. *JAMA* 1982; 247: 1448 – 1450.

[200] Norrby-Teglud A, Low DE, McGeer A, Kotb M. Superantigenic activity produced by group A streptococcal isolates is neutralized by plasma from IVIG-treated streptococcal isolates is neutralized by plasma from IVIG-treated streptococcal toxic shock syndrome patients. *Adv Exp Med Biol* 1997; 418: 563 – 566.

[201] Fry DE. Toxic shock syndrome. In: *Surgical Infection*, Fry DE (Ed). Boston: Little Brown, 1995, pp 569 – 576.

[202] Sirinek KR. Diagnosis and treatment of intra-abdominal abscesses. *Surg Infect* 2000; 1: 31 - 38.

[203] Montgomery RS, Wilson SE. Intraabdominal abscesses: image-guided diagnosis and therapy. *Clin Infect Dis* 1996; 23: 28 – 36.

[204] Barkhausen J, Stoblen F, Dominguez-Fernandez E, Henseke P, Muller RD. Impact of CT in patients with sepsis of unknown origin. *Acta Radiol* 1999; 40: 552 -555.

[205] Lal NR, Kazerooni EA, Bree RL. Development and implementation of an appropriateness guideline for use of CT in cases of suspected intraabdominal abscess. *Acad Radiol* 2000; 7: 711 – 716.

[206] Levison MA. Percutaneous versus open operative drainage of intra-abdominal abscesses. *Infect Dis Clin North Am* 1992; 6: 525 - 544.

[207] Khurrum Baig M, Hua Zhao R, Batista O, et al. Percutaneous postoperative intra-abdominal abscess drainage after elective colorectal surgery. *Tech Coloproctol* 2002; 6:159-164.

[208] Marano I, Mainenti PP, Selva G, et al. Computerized tomography-guided drainage of postoperative abdominal fluid collections. *Radiol Med* 1999; 97: 160 - 165.
[209] Bufalari A, Giustozzi G, Moggi L. Postoperative intraabdominal abscesses: percutaneous versus surgical treatment. *Acta Chir Belg* 1996; 96:197-200.
[210] Thanos L, Dailiana T, Papaioannou G, et al. Percutaneous CT-guided drainage of splenic abscess. *AJR Am J Roentgenol* 2002;179: 629 –632.
[211] Lankisch PG, Pflichthofer D, Lehnick D. No strict correlation between necrosis and organ failure in severe acute pancreatitis. *Pancreas* 2000; 20: 319 – 322.
[212] Bassi C, Falconi M, Girelli F, et al. Microbiological findings in severe pancreatitis. *Surg Res Commun* 1989; 5: 1 – 4.
[213] Isenmann R, Rau B, Beger HG. Bacterial infection and extent of necrosis are determinants of organ failure in patients with acute necrotizing pancreatitis. *Br J Surg* 1999; 86: 1020 – 1024.
[214] Gloor B, Muller CA, Worni M, et al. Late mortality in patients with severe acute pancreatitis. *Br J Surg* 2001; 88: 975 – 979.
[215] Banks PA, Gerzof SG, Langevin RE, et al. CT-guided aspiration of suspected pancreatic infection: bacteriology and clinical outcome. *Int J Pancreatol* 1995; 18: 265 – 270.
[216] British Society of Gastroenterology: United Kingdom guidelines for the management of acute pancreatitis. *Gut* 1998; 42 (Suppl 2): S1 – S13.
[217] Uhl W, Warshaw A, Imrie C, et al. IAP guidelines for the surgical management of acute pancreatitis. *Pancreatology* 2002; 2: 565 – 573.
[218] Widdison AL, Karanjia ND. Pancreatic infection complicating acute pancreatitis. *Br J Surg* 1993; 80: 148 – 154.
[219] Buchler MW, Gloor B, Muller CA, et al. Acute necrotizing pancreatitis Treatment stragegy according to the status of infection. *Ann Surg* 2000; 232: 619 – 626.
[220] Fernandez-del Castillo C, Rattner DW, Makary MA, et al. Debridement and closed packing for the treatment of necrotizing pancreatitis. *Ann Surg* 1998; 228: 676 – 684.
[221] Sarr MG, Nagorney DM, Mucha PJ, et al. Acute necrotizing pancreatitis: Management by planned, staged pancreatic necrosectomy / debridement and delayed primary wound closure over drains. *Br J Surg* 1991; 78: 576 – 581.
[222] Tenner S, Sica G, Hughes M, et al. Relationship of necrosis to organ failure in severe acute pancreatitis. *Gastroenterology* 1997; 113: 899 – 903.
[223] Rau B, Pralle U, Uhl W, et al. Management of sterile necrosis in instances of severe acute pancreatitis. *J Am Coll Surg* 1995; 181: 279 – 288.

[224] Hartwing W, Maksan SM, Foitzik T, et al. Reduction in mortality with delayed surgical therapy of severe pancreatitis. *J Gastrointest Surg* 2002; 6: 481 – 487.

[225] Kivilaakso E, Fraki O, Nikki P, Lempinen M. Resection of the pancreas for acute fulminant pancreatitis. *Surg Gynecol Obstet* 1981; 152: 493 – 498.

[226] Mier J, Leon EL, Castillo A, et al. Early versus late necrosectomy in severe necrotizing pancreatitis. *Am J Surg* 1997; 173: 71 – 75.

[227] Baron TH, Thaggard WG, Morgan DE, Stanley RJ. Endoscopic therapy for organized pancreatic necrosis. *Gastroenterology* 1996; 111: 755 – 764.

[228] Carter CR, McKay CJ, Imrie CW. Percutaneous necrosectomy and sinus tract endoscopy in the management of infected pancreatic necrosis; an initial experience. *Ann Surg* 2000; 232: 175 – 180.

[229] Tsiotos GG, Luque-de LE, Soreide JA, et al. Management of necrotizing pancreatitis by repeated operative necrosectomy using a zipper technique. *Am J Surg* 1998; 175: 91 – 98.

[230] Schierholz JM, Beuth J. Implant infections: a haven for opportunistic bacteria. *J Hosp Infect* 2001; 49: 87-93.

[231] von Eiff C, Peters G, Heilmann C. Pathogenesis of infections due to coagulase-negative staphylococci. *Lancet Infect Dis* 2002; 2: 677 - 685.

[232] Vandecasteele SJ, Van Wijngaerden E, Van Eldere J, Peetermans WE. New insights in the pathogenesis of foreign body infections with coagulase negative staphylococci. *Acta Clin Belg* 2000; 55: 148 - 153.

[233] Maki DG, Weise CE, Sarafin HW. A semiquantitative culture method for identifying intravenous catheter-related infection. *N Engl J Med* 1977; 296: 1305 – 1309.

[234] Sherertz RJ, Heard SO, Raad II. Diagnosis of triple-lumen catheter infection: comparison of roll-plate, sonication, and flushing methodologies. *J Clin Microbiol* 1997; 35: 641 – 646.

[235] Cook DJ, Randolph A, Kernerman P, et al. Central venous catheter replacement strategies: a systemic review of the literature. *Crit Care Med* 1997; 25: 1417 – 1424.

[236] Maki D, Stolz S, Wheeler S, Mermel LA. Prevention of central venous catheter-related blood-stream infection by use of an antiseptic-impregnated catheter. *Ann Intern Med* 1997; 127: 257 – 266.

[237] Clarke DE, Raffin TA. Infectious complications of indwelling long-term central venous catheters. *Chest* 1990; 97: 966 – 972.

[238] Murray CK, Beckius ML, McAllister K. Fusarium proliferatum superficial suppurative thrombophlebitis. *Mil Med* 2003; 168: 426 - 427.

[239] Timsit JF. Scheduled replacement of central venous catheters is not necessary. *Infect Control Hosp Epidemiol* 2000; 21: 371 - 374.

[240] Bregenzer T, Conen D, Sakmann P, Widmer AF. Is routine replacement of peripheral intravenous catheters necessary? *Arch Intern Med* 1998; 158: 151 – 156.

[241] Gajic O, Urrutia LE, Sewani H, et al. Acute abdomen in the medical intensive care unit. *Crit Care Med* 2002; 30: 1187 – 1190.

[242] Kollef MH, Allen BT. Determinants of outcome for patients in the medical intensive care unit requiring abdominal surgery: a prospective, single-center study. *Chest* 1994; 106: 1822 – 1828.

[243] Gregor P, Prodger JD. Mead Johnson Critical Care Symposium for the Practicing Surgeon. Abdominal Crisis in the Intensive Care Unit. *Can J Surg* 1988; 31: 331 – 332.

[244] Stapakis JC, Thickman D. Diagnosis of pneumoperitoneum: abdominal CT vs. upright chest film. *J Comput Assist Tomogr* 1992; 16: 713 – 716.

[245] Jacobs JE, Birnbaum BA. Abdominal computed tomography of intensive care unit patients. *Semin Roentgenol* 1997; 32: 128 – 141.

[246] Boland GW, Slater G, Lu DS, et al. Prevalence and significance of gallbladder abnormalities seen on sonography in intensive care unit patients. *AJR Am J Roentgenol* 2000; 174: 973 – 977.

[247] Walsh RM, Popocivh MJ, Hoadley J. Bedside diagnostic laparoscopy and peritoneal lavage in the intensive care unit. *Surg Endosc* 1998; 12: 1405 – 1409.

[248] Byrne MF, Suhocki P, Mitchell RM, et al. Percutaneous cholecystostomy in patients with acute cholecystitis: experience of 45 patients at a US referral center. *J Am Coll Surg* 2003; 197: 206-211.

[249] Akhan O, Akinci D, Ozmen MN. Percutaneous cholecystostomy. *Eur J Radiol* 2002; 43: 229 - 236.

[250] Gouma DJ. Management of acute cholangitis. *Dig Dis* 2003; 21: 25 - 29.

[251] Gedebou TM, Wong RA, Rappaport WD, Jaffe P, Kahsai D, Hunter GC. Clinical presentation and management of iatrogenic colon perforations. *Am J Surg* 1996; 172: 454 – 458.

[252] Jentschura D, Raute M, Winter J, et al. Complications in endoscopy of the lower gastrointestinal tract. Therapy and Prognosis. *Surg Endosc* 1994; 8: 672 – 676.

[253] Liolios A, Oropello JM, Benjamin E. Gastrointestinal complications in the intensive care unit. *Clin Chest Med* 1999; 20: 329 – 324.

[254] Polk HC, Shields CL. Remote organ failure: a valid sign of occult intraabdominal infection. *Surgery* 1977; 81: 310 – 313.

[255] Fry DE, Pearlstein L, Fulton RL, Polk HC. Multiple system organ failure: the role of uncontrolled infection. *Arch Surg* 1980; 115: 136 – 140.
[256] Ferraris VA. Exploratory laparotomy for potential abdominal sepsis in patients with multiple organ failure. *Arch Surg* 1983; 118: 1130 – 1133.
[257] Bunt TJ. Non-directed relaparotomy for intraabdominal sepsis; a futile procedure. *Am Surg* 1986; 52: 294 – 298.
[258] Grant JP. Nutritional support in critically ill patients. *Ann Surg* 1994; 220: 610 – 616.
[259] Moore FA, Feliciano DV, Andrassy RJ, et al. Early enteral feeding, compared with parenteral, reduces postoperative septic complications; the results of a meta-analysis. *Ann Surg* 1992; 216: 172 – 183.
[260] Kudsk KA, Stone JM, Carpenter G, Sheldon GF. Enteral and parenteral feeding influences mortality after hemoglobin E. Coli peritonitis in normal rats. *J Trauma* 1983; 23: 605 – 609.
[261] Kudsk KA. Gut mucosal nutritional support. Enteral nutrition as primary therapy after multiple system trauma. *Gut* 1994; 35 (Suppl 1); S52 – S54.
[262] Sakorafas GH, Krespis EN. Methods of enteral nutrition. *Iatriki* 1992, 61: 482 – 491 (GR).
[263] Sakorafas GH. Enteral nutrition in Surgery. *Hell Armed Forces Med Rev* 1992, 26: 129 - 148.
[264] Cerra FB, Benitez MR, Blackburn GL, et al. Applied nutrition in ICU patients; a consensus statement of the American College of Chest Physicians. *Chest* 1997; 111: 769 – 778.
[265] Singh G, Harkema JM, Mayberry AJ, Chaudry IH. Severe depression of gut absorptive capacity in patients following trauma or sepsis. *J Trauma* 1994; 36: 803 – 809.
[266] Singh G, Chaudry KI, Chudler LC, Chaudry IH. Sepsis produces early depression of gut absorptive capacity restoration with diltiazem treatment. *Am J Physiol* 1992; 263: R19 – 23.
[267] Long C. Metabolic response to injury and illness. Estimation of energy and protein needs from indirect calorimetry and nitrogen balance. *JPEN J Parenter Enter Nutr* 1979; 3: 452 – 456.
[268] McCarthy MC. Nutritional support in the critically ill surgical patient. *Surg Clin North Am* 1991; 71: 831 – 841.
[269] Kalfarentzos J. *Nutritional support. Monograph*, Litsas (Ed), Athens 1986, pp 1 – 130.
[270] Clevenger FW. Nutritional support in the patient with the systemic inflammatory response syndrome. *Am J Surg* 1993; 165 (2A Suppl): 68S – 74S.

[271] Koretz RL. Nutritional supplementation in the ICU: how critical is nutrition for the critically ill? *Am J Respir Crit Care Med* 1995; 151: 570 – 573.

[272] Glauser MP. Pathophysiologic basis of sepsis; considerations for future strategies of intervention. *Crit Care Med* 2000; 28 (Suppl): S4 – S8.

[273] Neugebauer E, Rixen D, Raum M, Schafer U. Thirty years of anti-mediator treatment in sepsis and septic shock: What have we learned? *Langenbecks Arch Surg* 1998; 383: 26 – 34.

[274] Zeni F, Freeman B, Natanson C. Anti-inflammatory therapies to treat sepsis and septic shock: a reassessment. *Crit Care Med* 1997; 25: 1095 – 1100.

[275] Kox WJ, Volk T, Kox SN, Volk HD. Immunomodulatory therapies in sepsis. *Intensive Care Med* 2000; 26: S124 – S128.

[276] Abraham E, Anzueto A, Cutierrez G, et al. Double-blind randomised controlled trial of monoclonal antibody to human tumor necrosis factor in treatment of septic shock. *Lancet* 1998; 351: 929 – 933.

[277] Bone RC, Balk RA, Fein AM, et al. A second large controlled study of E5, a monoclonal antibody to endotoxin: results of a prospective, multicenter, randomised, controlled trial. *Crit Care Med* 1995; 23: 994 – 1006.

[278] Angus DC, Birmingham D, Balk RA, et al. E5 murine monoclonal antiendotoxin antibody in gram-negative sepsis: a randomized controlled trial. E5 Study Investigators. JAMA 2000; 283:1723- 1730.

[279] Hotchkiss RS, Karl IE. The pathophysiology and treatment of sepsis. *N Engl J Med* 2003; 348: 138 – 150.

[280] Czermak BJ, Sarma V, Pierson CL, et al. Protective effects of C5a blockade in sepsis. *Nat Med* 1999; 5: 788 – 792.

[281] Guo RF, Huber-Lang M, Wang X, et al. Protective effects of anti-C5a in sepsis-induced thymocyte apoptosis. *J Clin Invest* 2000; 106: 1271 – 1280.

[282] Huber Lang MS, Sarma JV, McGuire SR et al. Protective effects of anti-C5a peptide antibodies in experimental sepsis. *FASEB J* 2001; 15: 568 – 570.

[283] Rogiers P. Hemofiltration treatment for sepsis; is it time for controlled trials? *Kidney Int* 1999: 56 (Suppl 72): S99 – S103.

[284] Gotloid L, Shostak A, Lev A, Fudin R, Jaichenko J. Treatment of surgical and non-surgical septic multiorgan failure with bicarbonate hemodialysis and sequential hemofiltration. *Intensive Care Med* 1995; 21: 104 – 111.

[285] Bellomo R, Balwin I, Cole Ronco C. Preliminary experience with high-volume hemofiltration in human septic shock. *Kidney Int* 1998; 54 (Suppl 66): S182 – S185.

[286] Boulain T, Delpech M, Legras A, et al. Continuous venovenous hemofiltration in acute renal failure associated with multiple organ failure: influence on outcome. *Clin Intens Care* 1996; 7: 4 – 10.

[287] Schiffl H, Lang SM, Fischer R. Daily hemodialysis and the outcome of acute renal failure. *N Engl J Med* 2002; 346: 305 – 310.

[288] Kollef MH. Opinion: the clinical use of selective digestive decontamination. *Crit Care* 2000;4: 327-332.

[289] Bonten MJ, Kullberg BJ, van Dalen R, et al. Selective digestive decontamination in patients in intensive care. The Dutch Working Group on Antibiotic Policy. *J Antimicrob Chemother* 2000;46: 351-362.

[290] Sprung CL, Caralis PV, Marcial EH, et al. The effects of high-dose corticosteroids in patients with septic shock. *N Engl J Med* 1984; 311: 1137 – 1143.

[291] Cronin L, Cook DJ, Carlet J, et al. Corticosteroid treatment for sepsis; a critical reappraisal and meta-analysis of the literature. *Crit Care Med* 1995; 23: 1430 – 1439.

[292] Annane D, Sebille V, Charpentier C, et al. Effect of treatment with low doses of hydrocortisone and fludrocortisone on mortality in patients with septic shock. *JAMA* 2002; 288: 862-871.

[293] Briegel J, Forst H, Haller M, et al. Stress doses of hydrocortisone reverse hyperdynamic septic shock; a prospective, randomized, double blind, single-center study. *Crit Care Med* 1999; 27: 723 – 732.

[294] Boellaert PE, Charpentier C, Levy B, Debouverie M, Audibert G, Larcan A. Reversal of late septic shock with supra-physiologic doses of hydrocortisone. *Crit Care Med* 1998; 26: 645 – 650.

[295] Spijkstra JJ, Girbes ARJ. The continuing story of corticosteroids in the treatment of septic shock. *Intensive Care Med* 2000; 26: 496 – 500.

[296] Annane D. Corticosteroids for septic shock. *Crit Care Med* 2001; 29 (Suppl): S117 – S120.

[297] Zaloga GP. Sepsis-induced adrenal deficiency syndrome. *Crit Care Med* 2001; 29: 688 – 690.

[298] Shenker Y, Skatrud JB. Adrenal insufficiency in critically ill patients. *Am J Respir Crit Care Med* 2001; 163: 1520 – 1523.

[299] Annane D, Sebille V, Troche G, Raphael JC, Gajdos P, Bellissant E. A 3-level prognostic classification in septic shock based on cortisol levels and cortisol response to corticotrophin. *JAMA* 2000; 283: 1038 – 1045.

[300] Abraham E, Evans T. Corticosteroids and septic shock. *JAMA* 2002; 288: 886 – 887.

[301] Arons MM, Wheeler AP, Bernard GR, et al. Effects of ibuprofen on the physiology and survival of hypothermic sepsis. Ibuprofen in Sepsis Study Group. *Crit Care Med* 1999; 27: 699-707.

[302] Bernard GR, Wheeler AP, Russell JA, et al. Effects of ibuprofen on the physiology and survival of patients with sepsis. *N Engl J Med* 1997; 336: 912 – 918.

[303] Bernard GR, Vincent JL, Laterre PF, et al. Efficacy and safety of recombinant human activated protein C for severe sepsis. *N Engl J Med* 2001; 344: 699 – 709.

[304] Matthay MA. Severe sepsis – a new treatment with both anticoagulant and anti-inflammatory properties. *N Engl J Med* 2001; 344: 759 – 762.

[305] Joyce DE, Gelbert L, Ciaccia A, et al. Gene expression profile on antithrombotic protein C defines new mechanisms modulating inflammation and apoptosis. *J Biol Chem* 2001; 276: 11199 – 11203.

[306] Cohen J, Guyatt G, Bernard GR, et al. New strategies for clinical trials in patients with sepsis and septic shock. *Crit Care Med* 2001; 29: 880 – 886.

[307] Quartin AA, Schein RM, Kett DH, Peduzzi PN. Magnitude and duration on the effect of sepsis on survival. Department of Veterans Affairs Systemic Sepsis Cooperative Studies Group. *JAMA* 1997; 277: 1058 – 1063.

[308] Warren HS, Suffredini AF, Eichacker PQ, Munford RS. Risks and benefits of activated protein C treatment for severe sepsis. *N Engl J Med* 2002; 347: 1027 – 1030.

[309] Manns BJ, Lee H, Doig CJ, Johnson D, Donaldson C. An economic evaluation of activated protein C for severe sepsis. *N Engl J Med* 2002; 347: 993 – 1000.

[310] Siegel JP. Assessing the use of activated protein C in the treatment of severe sepsis. *N Engl J Med* 2002; 347: 1030 – 1034.

[311] Levi M, Jonge E, Poll T. Rational for restoration of physiological anticoagulant pathways in patients with sepsis and disseminated intravascular coagulation. *Crit Care Med* 2001; 29 (Suppl 7): S90 – S94.

[312] Baudo F, Caimi TM, de Cataldo F, et al. Antithrombin III (ATIII) replacement therapy in patients with sepsis and / or post-surgical complications: a controlled double-blind, randomised, multicenter study. *Intensive Care Med* 1998; 24: 336 – 342.

[313] Eisele B, Lamy M, Thijs LG, et al. Antithrombin III in patients with severe sepsis: a randomised, placebo-controlled, double-blind multicenter trial plus a meta-analysis on all randomised, placebo-controlled, double-blind trials with antithrombin III in severe sepsis. *Intensive Care Med* 1998; 24: 663 – 672.

[314] Bregengard C, Nordfang O, Wildoose P, Svendsen O, Hedner U, Diness V. The effect of two-domain tissue factor pathway inhibitor on endotoxin-induced disseminated intravascular coagulation in rabbits. *Blood Coagul Fibrinolysis* 1993; 4: 699 – 706.

[315] Elsayed YA, Nakagawa K, Kamikubo YI, et al. Effects of recombinant human tissue factor pathway inhibitor on thrombus formation and its in vivo distribution in a rat DIC model. *Am J Clin Pathol* 1996; 106: 574 – 583.

[316] Inthorn D, Hoffman JN, Hartl WH, et al. Antithrombin III supplementation in severe sepsis: beneficial effects on organ dysfunction. *Shock* 1997; 8: 328 – 334.

[317] Van de Berghe G, Wouters P, Weekers F, et al. Intensive insulin therapy in critically ill patients. *N Engl J Med* 2001; 345: 1359 – 1367.

[318] Go F, Gao E, Yue TL, et al. Nitric oxide mediates the antiapoptotic effect of insulin in myocardial ischemia-reperfusion: the roles of PI3-kinase, Akt, and endothelial nitric oxide synthase phosphorylation. *Circulation* 2002; 105: 1497 – 1502.

[319] Mutunga M, Fulton B, Bullock R, et al. Circulating endothelial cells in patients with septic shock. *Am J Respir Crit Care Med* 2001; 163: 195 – 200.

[320] Baudouin S. *Sepsis therapies: options for the future: endothelial cell replacement.* Program and abstracts of the 23rd International Symposium on Intensive Care and Emergency Medicine; March 18 – 21, 2003, Brussels, Belgium.

[321] Oberholzer C, Oberholzer A, Clare-Salzler M, Moldawer LL. Apoptosis in sepsis: a new target for therapeutic intervention. *FASEB J* 2001; 15: 879 – 892.

[322] Oberholzer C, Oberholzer A, Bahjat FR, et al. Targeted adenovirus-induced expression of IL-10 decreases thymic apoptosis and improves survival in murine sepsis. *Proc Natl Acad Sci USA* 2001; 98: 11503 – 11508.

[323] Hotchkiss RS, Tinsley KW, Swanson PE, et al. Prevention of lymphocyte cell death in sepsis improves survival in mice. *Proc Natl Acad Sci USA* 1999; 96: 14541 – 14546.

[324] Hotchkiss RS, Chang KC, Swanson PE, et al. Caspace inhibitors improve survival in sepsis; a critical role of the lymphocyte. *Nat Immunol* 2000; 1: 496 – 501.

[325] Coopersmith C, Stromberg PR, Dunne WM, et al. Inhibition of intestinal epithelial apoptosis and survival in a murine model of pneumonia-induced sepsis. *JAMA* 2002; 287: 1716 – 1721.

[326] Anel RL, Kumar A. Experimental and emerging therapies for sepsis and septic shock. *Expert Opin Investig Drugs* 2001;10: 1471-1485.

[327] Herndon DN, Ramzy PI, DebRoy MA, et al. Muscle protein catabolism after severe burn: effects of IGF-1 / IGFBP-3 treatment. *Ann Surg* 1999; 229: 713 – 719.

[328] Sakurai Y, Aarsland A, Herndon DN, et al. Stimulation of muscle protein synthesis by long-term insulin infusion in severely burned patients. *Ann Surg* 1995; 222: 283 – 294.

[329] Ziegler TR, Gatzen C, Wilmore DW. Strategies for attenuating protein-catabolic responses in the critically ill. *Ann Rev Med* 1994; 45: 459 – 464.

[330] Wilmore DW. The effect of glutamine supplementation in patients following elective surgery and accidental injury. *J Nutr* 2001; 131(9 Suppl): S2543 - S2551.

[331] Zaloga GB, Roberts P. Permissive underfeeding. *New Horiz* 1994; 2:257-263.

[332] Hotchkiss RS, Tinsley KW, Swanson PE, et al. Sepsis-induced apoptosis causes progressive profound depletion of B and CD4+ lymphocytes in humans. *J Immunol* 2001; 166: 6952 – 6963.

[333] Zeni F, Freeman BF, Natanson C. Anti-inflammatory therapies to treat sepsis and septic shock: a reassessment. *Crit Care Med* 1997; 25: 1095 – 1100.

[334] Oberholzer A, Oberholzer C, Moldawer LL. Sepsis syndromes; understanding the role of innate and acquired immunity. *Shock* 2001; 16: 83 – 96.

[335] Docke WD, Randow F, Syrbe U, et al. Monocyte deactivation in septic patients: restoration by IFN-gamma treatment. *Nat Med* 1997; 3: 678 – 681.

[336] O'Suilleabhain C, O'Sullivan ST, Kelly JL, et al. Interleukin-12 treatment restores normal resistance to bacterial challenge after burn injury. *Surgery* 1996; 120: 290 – 296.

[337] Caladra T, Echtenacher B, Roy DL, et al. Protection from septic shock by neutralization of macrophage migration inhibitory factor. *Nat Med* 2000; 6: 164 – 170.

[338] Werdan K. Pathophysiology of septic shock and multiple organ dysfunction syndrome and various therapeutic approaches with special emphasis on immunoglobulins. *Ther Apher* 2001; 5: 115 – 122.

[339] Werdan K. Supplemental immune globulins in sepsis. *Clin Chem Lab Med* 1999; 37: 341 – 349.

[340] Pilz G, Fateh-Moghadam S, Viell B, et al. Supplemental immunoglobulin therapy in sepsis and septic shock. *Theor Surg* 1993; 8: 61 – 83.

[341] Pilz G, Fraunberger P, Appel R, et al. Early prediction of outcome in score-identified, post-cardiac patients at high risk for sepsis, using soluble tumor necrosis factor receptor-p55 concentrations. *Crit Care Med* 1996; 24: 596 – 600.

[342] Pilz G, Appel R, Kreuzer E, Werdan K. Comparison of early Igm-enriched immunoglobulin vs polyvalent IgG administration in score-identified post-cardiac surgical patients at high-risk for sepsis. *Chest* 1997; 111: 419 – 426.

[343] Society of Critical Care Medicine: Pulmonary artery catheter consensus conference: Consensus Statement. *Crit Care Med* 1997; 25: 910.

[344] Hameed SM, Cohn SM. Gastric tonometry: the role of mucosal pH measurement in the management of trauma. *Chest.* 2003; 123(5 Suppl): 475S-481S.

[345] Martini L, Giavaresi G, Fini M, et al. Hemodynamic indices versus gastric tonometric measurements for prognosis of hemorrhagic shock: a porcine model. *Comp Med* 2003; 53:178 - 185.

[346] Bakker J, Coffernils M, Leon M, et al. Blood lactate levels are superior to oygen-derived variables in predicting outcome in septic shock. *Chest* 1991; 99: 956 – 962.

[347] Husain FA, Martin MJ, Mullenix PS, et al. Serum lactate and base deficit as predictors of mortality and morbidity. *Am J Surg* 2003; 185: 485 - 491.

[348] Krishnagopalan S, Kumar A, Parrillo JE, Kumar A. Myocardial dysfunction in the patient with sepsis. *Curr Opin Crit Care* 2002; 8: 376 –388.

[349] Grocott-Mason RM, Shah AM. Cardiac dysfunction in sepsis: new theories and clinical implications. *Intensive Care Med.* 1998; 24:286 - 295.

[350] Aube H, Milan C, Blettery B. Risk factors for septic shock in the early management of bacteremia. *Am J Med* 1992; 93: 283 – 289.

[351] Barriere S, Lowry S. An overview of mortality risk prediction in sepsis. *Crit Care Med* 1995; 23: 376 – 379.

[352] Marsh CB, Wewers MD. The pathogenesis of sepsis; factors that modulate the response to gram-negative bacterial infection. *Clin Chest Med* 1996; 17: 183 – 193.

[353] Marshall JC, Cook DJ, Christou NV, et al. Multiple organ dysfunction score: a reliable descriptor of a complex clinical outcome. *Crit Care Med* 1995; 23: 1638 – 1652.

[354] Vincent J-L, Moreno R, Takala J, et al. The SOFA (Sepsis-related Organ Failure Assessment) score to describe organ dysfunction/failure. *Intensive Care Med* 1996; 22: 707 – 710.

[355] Cook R, Cook DJ, Tilley J, et al. Multiple organ dysfunction: baseline and serial component scores. *Crit Care Med* 2001; 29: 2046 – 2050.

[356] Quartin AA, Schein RM, Kett DH, et al. Magnitude and duration on the effect of sepsis on survival. Department of Veterans Affairs Systemic Sepsis Cooperative Studies Group. *JAMA* 1997; 277: 1058 – 1063.

[357] Kreger BE, Craven DE, McCabe WR. Gram-negative bacteremia. IV. Re-evaluation of clinical features and treatment in 612 patients. *Am J Med* 1980; 68: 344 – 355.

[358] Renaud B, Brun-Buisson C, ICU-bacteremia Study Group: Outcomes of primary and catheter-related bacteremia: A cohort and case-control study in critically ill patients. *Am J Respir Crit Care Med* 2001; 163: 1584 – 1590.

[359] Glauser MP, Zanetti G, Baumgartner JD, et al. Septic shock: Pathogenesis. *Lancet* 1991; 9: 1220 – 1222.

[360] Hausfater P, Garric S, Ayed SB, et al. Usefulness of procalcitonin as a marker of systemic infection in emergency department: a prospective study. *Clin Infect Dis* 2002; 34: 895 – 901.

[361] Damas P, Ledoux D, Dys M, et al. Cytokine serum level during severe sepsis in human IL-6 as a marker of severity. *Ann Surg* 1992; 215: 356 – 362.

[362] Panacek EA, Kaul M. IL-6 as a marker of excessive TNF-alpha activity in sepsis. *Sepsis* 1999; 3: 65 – 73.

[363] Doglio GR, Pusajo JF, Egurrola MA, et al. Gastric mucosal pH as a prognostic index of mortality in critically ill patients. *Crit Care Med* 1991; 19: 1037 – 1040.

[364] Le Gall JR, Lemeshow S, Leleu G, et al. Customized probability models for early severe sepsis in adult intensive care patients. *JAMA* 1995; 273: 644 – 650.

[365] Le Gall JR, Lemeshow S, Saulnier F. A new simplified acute physiology score (SAPS II) based on a European/North American multicenter study. *JAMA* 1993; 270: 2957 – 2963.

[366] Knaus WA, Draper EA, Wagner DP, et al. APACHE II: A severity of disease classification system. *Crit Care Med* 1985; 13: 818 – 825.

[367] Knaus WA, Wagner DP, Draper EA, et al. The APACHE III prognostic system: risk prediction of hospital mortality for critically ill hospitalized adults. *Chest* 1991; 100: 1619 – 1624.

[368] Lemeshow S, Teres D, Klar J, et al. Mortality probability models (MPM II) based on an international cohort of intensive care unit patients. *JAMA* 1993; 270: 2478 – 2483.

[369] Le Gall JR, Klar J, Lemeshow S, et al. The logistic organ dysfunction system: a new way to assess organ dysfunction in the intensive care unit. *JAMA* 1996; 276: 802 – 809.

[370] Vincent JL, Ferreira F, Moreno R. Scoring systems for assessing organ dysfunction and survival. *Crit Care Clin* 2000; 16: 353 – 366.
[371] Rivers E, Nguyen B, Havstad S, et al. Early goal-directed therapy in the treatment of severe sepsis and septic shock. *N Engl J Med* 2001; 345: 1368 – 1377.

Index

A

B

C

G

H

I

J

L

Q

R

S

T

U

V

W